ABO-incompatible Organ Transplantation from Japan

ABO-incompatible Organ Transplantation from Japan

Invited papers from the International Meeting at the 41st Annual Meeting of the Japan Society for Transplantation held in Niigata on 29 October 2005

Editor:

Kota Takahashi
Division of Urology
Department of Regenerative and Transplant Medicine
Graduate School of Medical and Dental Sciences
Niigata University
Asahimachi 1, Niigata 951-8510
JAPAN

ELSEVIER

2006

ELSEVIER B.V.
Radarweg 29
P.O. Box 211, 1000 AE Amsterdam
The Netherlands

ELSEVIER Inc.
525 B Street, Suite 1900
San Diego, CA 92101-4495
USA

ELSEVIER Ltd
The Boulevard, Langford Lane
Kidlington, Oxford OX5 1GB
UK

ELSEVIER Ltd
84 Theobalds Road
London WC1X 8RR
UK

First edition 2006

Library of Congress Cataloging in Publication Data
A catalog record is available from the Library of Congress.

British Library Cataloguing in Publication Data
A catalogue record is available from the British Library.

International Congress Series No. 1292
ISBN: 978-0-444-52165-1 / 0-444-52165-8
ISSN: 0531-5131

∞ The paper used in this publication meets the requirements of ANSI/NISO Z39.48-1992 (Permanence of Paper).
Printed in The Netherlands.

International Congress Series 1292 (2006) v

www.ics-elsevier.com

Preface

ABO-incompatible transplants and partial liver transplants from living donors can be cited as two procedures that can be conveyed to the world by Japan with confidence. Since the donation of cadaver organs is extremely rare in Japan, ironically, these transplants have become prevalent as a way of expanding the accommodation of transplants.

However, by performing these transplants, new findings that could not be uncovered through cadaver transplants have been revealed, making significant contributions to immunology and transplantations.

In Japan, more than 700 ABO-incompatible kidney transplants and over 300 ABO-incompatible liver transplants have been performed, and the results improve yearly. The mechanism of antibody-mediated rejection and accommodation that occur with the involvement of ABO blood types has been clarified, and the establishment of treatment strategies for immunosuppressive therapy based on the mechanism has led to the prevalence and improvement in the results of these transplants.

In 2005, I was blessed with the opportunity to organize the 41st Annual Meeting of the Japan Society for Transplantation. It was the chance of a lifetime to hold an international symposium on ABO-incompatible transplants, and in the same year, the 2nd Annual International ABO-Incompatible Transplantation Conference was held in Sweden. Holding these kinds of symposiums across the world has important implications, and I hope that ABO-incompatible transplants become more prevalent throughout the world as a result.

We invited the following doctors, who are active throughout the world in transplant surgery in this field, and requested them to give speeches at the recent symposium: Douglas W. Hanto (Massachusetts), Yuich Iwaki (California), Robert A. Montgomery (Maryland), Richard N. Pierson, III (Maryland), David H. Sachs (Massachusetts), Mark D. Stegall (Minnesota), Gunnar Tyden (Stockholm), Lori J. West (Toronto), and Kazuhiko Yamada (Massachusetts). Seizing this opportunity, the content of the speeches has been developed into a manuscript, which will be published by Elsevier's International Congress Series. This manuscript will become the bible of ABO-incompatible transplants, which I hope will lead to improvements in transplant results.

Professor Kota Takahashi, M.D. PhD.

0531-5131/ © 2006 Published by Elsevier B.V.
doi:10.1016/j.ics.2006.03.053

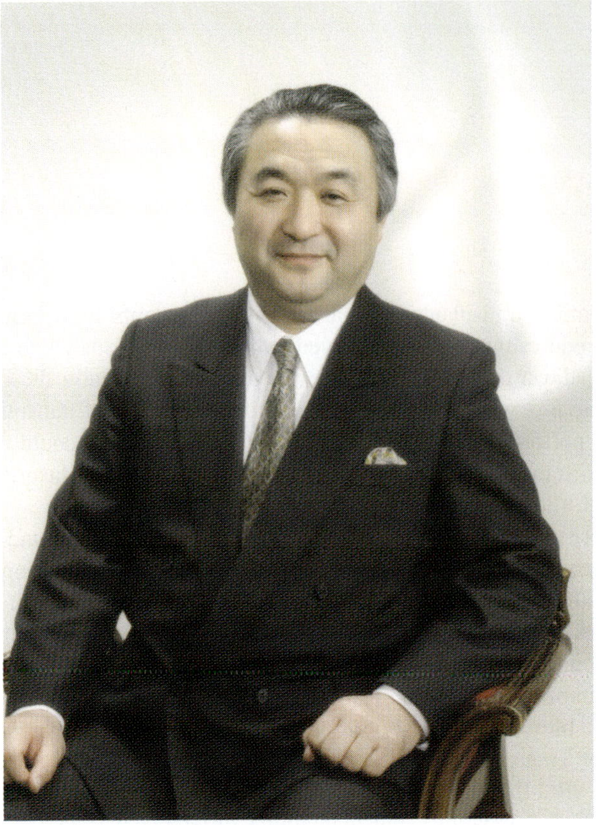

Prof. K. Takahashi

Contents

Preface v

Photo of Prof. K. Takahashi vi

Antigens and antibodies 1

Standardization of the assay method for anti-A/B antibody titers and its problems
T. Kobayashi 3

Donor-specific suppression of blood group antibodies in ABO-incompatible kidney transplantation
A. Aikawa, O. Takehiro, M. Yamashita, T. Kawamura, J. Inasaka, Y. Itabashi, K. Sakai, S. Mizuiri, T. Kanai, N. Kawada and A. Hasegawa 8

Severe rejection of rat intestinal grafts overexpressing human histo-blood group A/B transferase
S. Inoue, K. Tahara, J. Fujishiro, W. Zhou, H. Ohdan, T. Asahara, K. Hasnizume, M. Kaneko, Y. Hakamata, K. Takeuchi, S. Iwamoto and E. Kobayashi 13

Pathology 23

Correlation of conventional histology, clinical outcomes, and C4d immunostaining in ABO-incompatible liver transplantation
H. Haga, H. Sakashita, M.-C. Wen, A. Miyagawa-Hayashino, H. Egawa and T. Manabe 25

Kidney transplantation 33

ABO-incompatible kidney transplantation in Japan
K. Saito and K. Takahashi 35

Excellent long-term outcomes of ABO-incompatible kidney transplantation in children
S. Shishido, H. Asanuma, H. Satoh, M. Saneshige and Y. Nanpo 42

Liver transplantation 51

ABO-incompatible transplantation: Accommodation by upregulation of protective genes — A hypothesis
D.W. Hanto 53

Lung transplantation 61

ABO-incompatible lung transplantation
R.N. Pierson, J. Moore, R.M. Merion and A.M.I. Azimzadeh 63

Memorial lecture 71

A new immunosuppressive therapy in ABO-incompatible kidney transplantation based on a new concept of accommodation
K. Takahashi 73

Antibody removal 89

The safety measures for double filtration plasma apheresis (DFPP) before ABO-incompatible kidney transplantation
S. Nishi, S. Hasegawa, F. Gejyo, K. Saito, Y. Nakagawa and K. Takahashi 91

Rituximab 97

Newly developed preconditioning regimen consisting of rituximab, splenectomy and plasmapheresis for non-responders to conventional regimen in ABO-incompatible kidney transplantation
S. Teraoka, K. Kai, K. Iwato, Y. Kato, K. Nanmoku, A. Sannomiya, I. Koyama, T. Toujinbara, I. Nakajima and S. Fuchinoue 99

Prophylactic use of anti-CD20 monoclonal antibody in ABO-incompatible liver transplantation
M. Ueda, A. Yoshizawa, H. Haga, F. Oike, H. Egawa and K. Tanaka 105

Sensitization and preformed antibody-positive transplantation 111

Overcoming antibody barriers to transplantation: ABO-incompatible and positive cross-match kidney transplantation at Mayo Clinic – Rochester
M.D. Stegall 113

Xenotransplantation 121

GalT knockout pig to baboon xenotransplantation
K. Yamada and D.H. Sachs 123

Author index 129

Keyword index 131

Antigens and antibodies

ELSEVIER

International Congress Series 1292 (2006) 3–7

www.ics-elsevier.com

Standardization of the assay method for anti-A/B antibody titers and its problems

Takaaki Kobayashi *

Department of Surgery II, Nagoya University School of Medicine, 65 Tsurumai-cho, Showa-ku, Nagoya 466-8550, Japan

Abstract. Introduction of effective treatments such as (double filtration) plasmapheresis, splenectomy, intravenous immunoglobulin and potent immunosuppressive agents including anti-CD20 monoclonal antibody, has greatly improved graft outcome in ABO-incompatible transplantation. The measurement of anti-blood group A/B antibody titers is considered to be important, because it would provide useful information on prognosis and indication of transplantation, selection of treatments and prediction of acute rejection. Isohemagglutinin assay in serial-doubling dilutions of serum sample by tube test has been basically used in most institutions. However, detailed assay procedure seemed to vary between institutions. Furthermore, the determination by visual observation might cause a problem of inter-examiner variability. The Japanese ABO-Incompatible Transplantation Committee has conducted a series of nationwide surveys to assess the current status of inter-institutional variation in measurement of anti-A/B antibody titer. In the first survey, serum samples from 6 healthy volunteers with blood groups A ($n=2$), B ($n=2$) and O ($n=2$) were sent to 29 institutions where ABO-incompatible kidney or liver transplantation has been performed. Anti-A/B antibody titer was measured by its own protocol. Inter-institutional difference of measured values reached to 32-fold and 256-fold in IgM and IgG, respectively. As this variability was too wide for detailed analysis, the provisional standard protocol for the assay was determined according to the result of questionnaire survey. Next, 38 and 40 institutions participated in the second (in 2004) and the third survey (in 2005), respectively. Anti-A/B antibody titers of serum samples were measured by the standard procedure. Analysis of survey revealed that intra-institutional variation was reduced to below 8-fold (mostly 2- to 4-fold), although several institutions still needed some guidance. Standardization of the assay procedure and quality control survey would be necessary to improve the accuracy of measurement.

Abbreviations: RBC, red blood cells; DTT, dithiothreitol; 2ME, 2-mercaptoethanol.

* Tel.: +81 52 744 2507; fax: +81 52 744 2444.
E-mail address: takakoba@med.nagoya-u.ac.jp.

doi:10.1016/j.ics.2006.03.058

Significance of measurement of anti-A/B antibody titer in ABO-incompatible transplantation should be discussed after the result of multi-center study is obtained. © 2006 Published by Elsevier B.V.

Keywords: ABO-incompatible transplantation; Anti-A/B antibody titer; Survey; Inter-institutional variation

Promotion of living donor transplantation has been attempted to alleviate the chronic shortage of donor organs. To extend the number of living donor, it would be essential to overcome transplantation in recipients with preformed anti-donor antibody (e.g. cross-match-positive or ABO blood group incompatible transplantation) which was considered to be a contraindication because of poor prognosis.

ABO-incompatible transplantation has high risk of antibody-mediated rejection. Blood group A/B antigens expressed on endothelial cells in the graft are reacted with anti-A/B antibodies in recipients, which certainly causes complement and endothelial activation. Release of von Willebrand factor, upregulation of tissue factor and plasminogen activator inhibitor-1, and degradation of heparan sulfate proteoglycan most likely make endothelial cells acquire a procoagulant state. Procoagulation and platelet aggregation develop congestion, thrombi and hemorrhage in the graft, resulting in graft failure. Thus, there are four major factors which are involved in antibody-mediated rejection, namely blood group A/B antigen, anti-A/B antibody, complement and coagulation. Among these factors, only anti-A/B antibodies are variable and measurable.

The measurement of anti-A/B antibody titer is considered to provide beneficial information on prognosis of transplantation, prediction of acute rejection, selection of effective treatment and indication of procedure for antibody removal in particular, because the following questions have been raised: To what extent should antibody titer be reduced at the time of transplantation? How low and for how long should antibody titer be

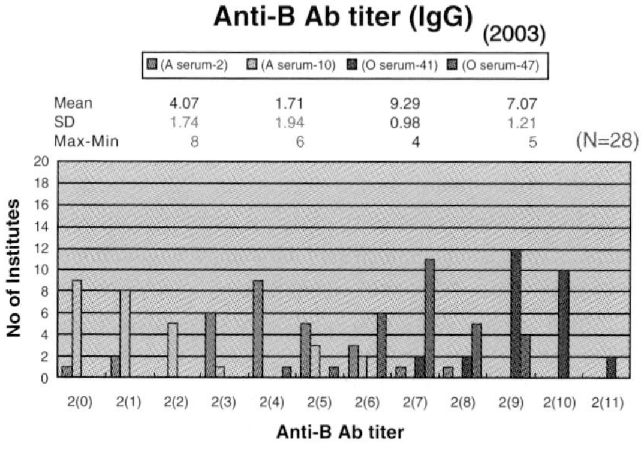

Fig. 1. Anti-B IgG antibody titer and number of institutions in the first survey conducted in 2003. The results of antibody titer measured in all institutions were described. Horizontal axis expresses antibody titers by a power of 2. The number of institutions is expressed on the vertical axis. Inter-institutional differences of measured IgG value between maximum and minimum titer reached 256-fold. As one institution measured only IgM titer, the total numbers of measured IgG titers were 28. The values of mean, S.D. and max–min are expressed by a power of 2.

Table 1
Provisional standard protocol (Japanese Society for ABO-I transplantation: 2003)

- ❑ Test tube methods
- ❑ RBC: commercially available or pooled; 3%
- ❑ RBC: serum sample=1:2 (e.g. 50 μL of RBC and 100 μL of serum)
- ❑ Centrifugation time: 15 s (5–60 s)

IgM assay using saline

- ❑ Room temperature (20–26 °C)
- ❑ Incubation time: 15 min

IgG assay using coombs

- ❑ Treatment of IgM: DTT (0.01M) (2ME sometimes showed insufficiency in IgM treatment)
- ❑ DTT: serum=1:1, 37 °C, 30 min (>60 min would possibly destroy IgG)
- ❑ No use of enhanced drug such as albumin or PEG
- ❑ Incubation time: 30 min
- ❑ Anti-human IgG (no use of non-specific Ab, e.g. anti-human IgG and complement)
- ❑ End point: + (not ±) in max dilution

maintained after transplantation? Is antibody removal necessary after transplantation, if so, what is the level of antibody titer?

For measuring anti-A/B antibody titer, there are several methods including isohemagglutinin assay in serial-doubling dilutions of serum using test tube, microplate or cassette (card) [1,2]. In addition, flow cytometry or ELISA can be also utilized [3]. Tube test is widely adopted in most institutes. However, tube test seems to contain several problems. Major problem is that tube test is based on visual observation, namely not objective but subjective judgment. Furthermore, some practice and experience would be necessary for technicians. It is likely that this would cause inter-examiner (technician) variation, resulting in inter-institutional variation. It must be a problem with unavailability of standard serum, degree of accuracy by semi-quantitative method (serial-doubling dilution) and discrimination between IgM and IgG antibody.

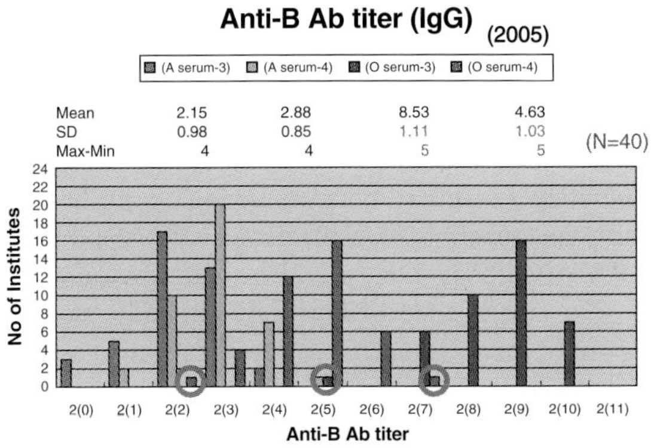

Fig. 2. Anti-B IgG antibody titer and number of institutions in the third survey conducted in 2005. The third survey was conducted using a provisional standard protocol in 40 collaborative institutions in 2005. Inter-institutional differences of measured IgG titer were reduced to below 8-fold, when the several institutions with large differences from the mean titer value which are indicated by circle, were removed.

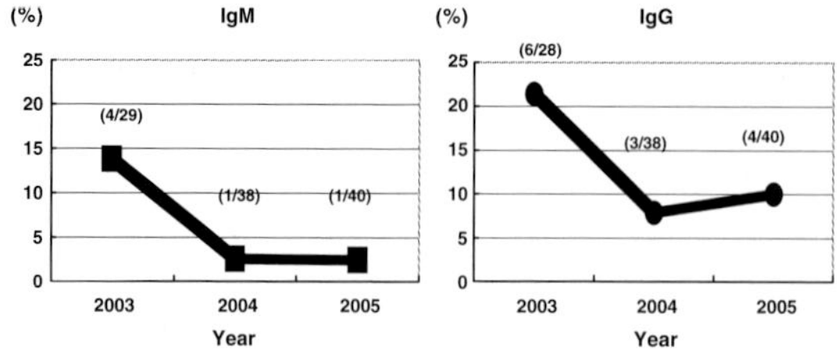

Fig. 3. Number of institutes which showed large difference from mean titer value. After the standard protocol for the measurement of anti-A/B antibody titer was introduced in 2004, the number of institutes which showed large difference (mean difference between measured titer and mean titer value >2 (1.25), namely 2 to the 1.25th power), was considerably reduced. However, for IgG measurement, 10% of institutes still had large difference from mean titer value.

A series of nationwide surveys were conducted by Japanese ABO-incompatible transplantation committee to assess inter-institutional variation in measurement of anti-A/B antibody titer. The results of surveys performed in 2003 and in 2004 were previously described [2]. Briefly, in the first survey in 2003, serum samples from 6 healthy volunteers with each two, blood group A, B, O, were sent to 29 collaborative institutions and anti-A/B antibody titer was measured by their customary methods. As the obtained results showed that inter-institutional difference reached 8- to 32-fold in IgM and 16- to 256-fold in IgG (Fig. 1), we attempted to standardize the assay. The provisional standard protocol was determined based on the result of the questionnaire survey (Table 1). Thirty-eight and forty institutions participated in the second (in 2004) and the third survey (in 2005), respectively. Anti-A/B antibody titers of serum samples were measured by the standard procedure. Analysis of the surveys revealed that intra-institutional variation was reduced to below 8-fold (mostly 2- to 4-fold), although several institutions which still had a large difference from the mean titer value might need some guidance (Fig. 2).

After the introduction of provisional standard protocol, the number of institutes which showed large difference from average titer value has been decreased (Fig. 3). For IgG measurement, approximately 10% of all collaborative institutes still had wide difference and seemed to require some guidance or training. As a task in the future, improvement of standard protocol, determination of gold standard in serum and periodical quality control survey might be essential.

Progress of treatments such as antibody removal, splenectomy, anti-metabolites, anti-CD20 monoclonal antibody and intravenous immunoglobulin has exactly improved the graft outcome of ABO-incompatible transplantation. We should examine whether the measurement of anti-A/B antibody titer would be really required, if so, how high its accuracy should be. The significance of anti A/B antibody titer should be elucidated through multi-center study, because each institute has only a small number of ABO-incompatible transplantations.

Acknowledgement

The author thanks all concerned people, especially the laboratory technicians of the following collaborative institutes in the Japanese ABO-Incompatible Transplantation

Committee; Doaikai Hakuai Hospital, Iwate Medical University, Ehime Prefectural Central Hospital, Ehime Prefectural Mishima Hospital, Osaka University, Osaka General Medical Center, Kanagawa Children's Medical Center, Gifu University, Kyoto University, Kyoto Prefectural University of Medicine, Japanese Red Cross Kumamoto Hospital, Gunma University, Keio University, Hiroshima Prefectural Hospital, Shizuoka Children's Hospital, Jichi Medical School, Chukyo Hospital, Sendai Shakaihoken Hospital, Tokyo Women's Medical University, Toho University, Tohoku University, Toyohashi Municipal Hospital, Nagoya University, Nagoya Daini Red Cross Hospital, Nara Medical University, Niigata University, Nippon Medical School, Hokkaido University, Mie University, Yokohama City University, Sunagawa City Medical Center, Okayama Medical Center, Saitama Medical School, Tokyo Medical University, Fujita Health University, Sapporo City General Hospital, Osaka Medical College, Tokyo Medical Center, Osaka Seamen's Insurance Hospital, SRL Inc., and the Olympus Corporation.

The author is also grateful to Drs. Junki Takamatsu and Koji Yamamoto, Transfusion Medicine, Nagoya University School of Medicine, for technical advice, and to Ms. Chieko Nakata, Ms. Yuko Miwa, Ms. Misao Niwa and Mr. Osamu Kamisawa for technical assistance.

References

[1] Technical manual committee, in: V. Vengelen-Tyler, K. Benson, D.R. Branch, et al. (Eds.), Technical manual, 12th ed., Bethesda; American Association of Blood Banks, 1996. Latest edition; In Brecher ME, ed. Technical manual 15th ed. Bethesda, American Association of Blood Banks, 2005.

[2] T Kobayashi, K Saito, A series of surveys on assay for anti-A/B antibody by Japanese ABO-incompatible transplantation committee, Xenotransplantation 13 (2006) 136–140.

[3] G. Stussi, et al., Isotype-specific detection of ABO blood group antibodies using a novel flow cytometric method, Br. J. Haematol. 130 (2005) 954–963.

International Congress Series 1292 (2006) 8–12

www.ics-elsevier.com

Donor-specific suppression of blood group antibodies in ABO-incompatible kidney transplantation

Atsushi Aikawa [a,*], Ohara Takehiro [b], Mioko Yamashita [a], Takeshi Kawamura [a], Jun Inasaka [a], Yoshihiro Itabashi [a], Ken Sakai [a], Sonoo Mizuiri [a], Tetsuo Kanai [c], Noriko Kawada [c], Akira Hasegawa [d]

[a] *Department of Nephrology, Toho University, 6-11-1, Omorinishi, Otaku, Tokyo, 143-8541, Japan*

[b] *Odawara Cardiovascular Hospital, Japan*

[c] *Division of Blood Transfusion, Toho University Omori Medical Center, Japan*

[d] *West Yokohama International General Hospital 6-11-1, Omorinishi Otaku, Tokyo, Japan #143-8541*

Abstract. *Purpose:* The aim of this study is to investigate the mechanism of long-term acceptance of ABO-incompatible renal allograft. *Methods:* Thirty-four ABO-incompatible kidney transplant recipients with blood group O were entered in this study. Eighteen and 16 recipients received a blood group B (B-to-O) and A1 (A1-to-O) allograft, respectively. Sixteen (O-to-O) recipients were control subjects. The titers of blood group antibodies were measured before pre-conditioning and following transplantation. Blood group antigens were stained in 32 graft biopsy specimen. *Results:* In 18 (B-to-O) and 16 (A1-to-O) recipients, only anti-B and anti-A1 antibodies, respectively, were significantly suppressed compared with those in 16 (O-to-O) more than 1 year post-transplantation. In eight (B-to-O) and seven (A1-to-O) recipients, only anti-B and anti-A1 antibodies, respectively, were significantly suppressed 1 year post-transplantation, compared with those pre-conditioning. Blood group antigens were stained with same intensity and pattern in any biopsy specimen under all conditions. There was no significant deposition of IgG and IgM in any biopsy specimen. These suggested that production of anti-donor blood group antibodies appeared to be specifically suppressed in long-term stable ABO-incompatible kidney transplant recipients. *Conclusion:* Accommodation of ABO-incompatible kidney transplantation could be explained by donor-specific blood group antibody suppression. © 2006 Elsevier B.V. All rights reserved.

Keywords: ABO-incompatible kidney transplantation; Blood group antibody; Blood group antigen

* Corresponding author. Tel.: +81 3 3762 4151; fax: +81 3 5471 3056.
E-mail address: aaikawa@med.toho-u.ac.jp (A. Aikawa).

0531-5131/
doi:10.1016/j.ics.2006.03.067

1. Introduction

ABO blood incompatible barrier can be crossed in kidney transplantation. Recently, we have obtained good clinical outcomes in ABO-incompatible kidney transplantation [1]. However, the mechanism of long-term acceptance of ABO-incompatible renal allograft, accommodation, has been clearly unknown. We noticed that anti-donor blood group antibodies (IgG and IgM) maintained the lower titers long-term post-transplantation in ABO-incompatible kidney transplantation [2]. The lower titers of blood group antibodies do not appear to react against donor blood group antigen that may result in accommodation. In the other hand, we do not know how long blood group antigens remain in the renal allograft. Herein, we investigated whether donor blood group antibodies were specifically suppressed for donor antigen in the ABO-incompatible kidney transplant recipients with blood group O. We also studied whether blood group antigens could express on acute rejection or under stable function in a renal allograft long-term post-transplantation.

2. Methods

Thirty-four ABO-incompatible kidney transplant recipients with blood group O were enrolled in this study. All these recipients maintained stable renal allograft function more than 1 year post-transplantation. Eighteen recipients were transplanted from a donor with blood group B (B-to-O) and 16 recipients were done from a donor with blood group A1 (A1-to-O). Sixteen recipients with blood group O transplanted from a donor with blood group O (O-to-O) were studied as control subjects. We also studied two recipients (A1 to O and B to O) who lost graft function due to delayed hyperacute rejection and chronic allograft nephropathy, respectively. Both the titers of anti-blood group antibodies (IgG and IgM) were measured serially pre-conditioning and following transplantation. All ABO-incompatible kidney transplant recipients were treated with plasmapheresis or exchange as pre-conditioning to reduce the anti-donor antibodies less than ×16. IgG was measured with albumin-Comb's method. IgM was initially pretreated with dithiothreitol and then measured with albumin-Comb's method. Blood group antigens (A1 and B) were stained with indirect immunoperoxidase method in 32 graft biopsy specimen, which included protocol biopsies 1 h ($n=8$), 2 months to 7 years post-transplant ($n=10$), acute cellular rejection ($n=11$) and acute humoral rejection ($n=3$). At the same time, IgG, IgM and complement components were also stained with immunofluorescent method.

Maintenance immunosuppression consisted of cyclosporine or tacrolimus, mycophenolate mofetil or azathioprine and methylprednisolone.

3. Results

The titers of anti-B IgG and IgM in 18 (B-to-O) were significantly lower than those of 16 (O-to-O), respectively ($p<0.0001$ and $p<0.0001$) (Table 1). However, the titers of anti-A1 IgG and IgM in 18 (B-to-O) did not differ from those of 16 (O-to-O). The titers of anti-A1 IgG and IgM in 16 (A1-to-O) were significantly lower than those of 16 (O-to-O), respectively ($p<0.01$ and $p<0.0001$) (Table 1). However, the titers

Table 1
Blood group antibodies more than 1 year post-transplantation

	N	Anti-B		Anti-A1	
		IgG	IgM	IgG	IgM
B-to-O	18	1.94 ± 1.66^{a}	1.39 ± 1.20^{a}	7.28 ± 1.27	5.94 ± 0.80
A1-to-O	16	5.00 ± 1.73	5.00 ± 0.91	2.31 ± 1.11^{b}	2.92 ± 1.70^{c}
O-to-O	16	6.07 ± 1.75	5.27 ± 1.03	6.93 ± 2.21	5.53 ± 1.27

Value=$\log_2 2^{n \pm \text{S.D}}$.
[a] $p<0.00001$, (B-to-O) compared with (O-to-O).
[b] $p<0.01$, (A1-to-O) compared with (O-to-O).
[c] $p<0.0001$, (A1-to-O) compared with (O-to-O).

of anti-B IgG and IgM did not differ from those of 16 (O-to-O). These demonstrated that only anti-donor blood group antibodies were specifically lower in (B-to-O) and (A1-to-O).

The titers of anti-B IgG and IgM 1 year post-transplantation were significantly lower than those pre-conditioning in eight (B-to-O), respectively ($p<0.0001$ and $p<0.00001$) (Fig. 1b,d). However, the titers of anti-A1 IgG and IgM 1 year post-transplantation did not differ from those pre-conditioning in 8 (B-to-O) (Fig. 1a,c). The titers of anti-A1 IgG and IgM 1 year post-transplantation were significantly lower than those pre-conditioning in seven (A1-to-O), respectively ($p<0.004$ and $p<0.009$) (Fig. 2a,c). However, the titers of anti-A1 IgG and IgM 1 year post-transplantation did not differ from those pre-conditioning in seven (A1-to-O) (Fig. 2b,d).

These also demonstrated that only anti-donor antibodies were specifically lower in (B-to-O) and (A1-to-O) 1 year post-transplantation.

In the recipient (A1-to-O) who had delayed hyperacute rejection, anti-A1 antibodies maintained the high titer (×2048) on rejection, after removal of allograft and then after ABO-compatible retransplantation under immunosuppression. In contrast, the recipient who failed graft function due to chronic allograft nephropathy, maintained low titer (<×32) after reintroduction to hemodialysis.

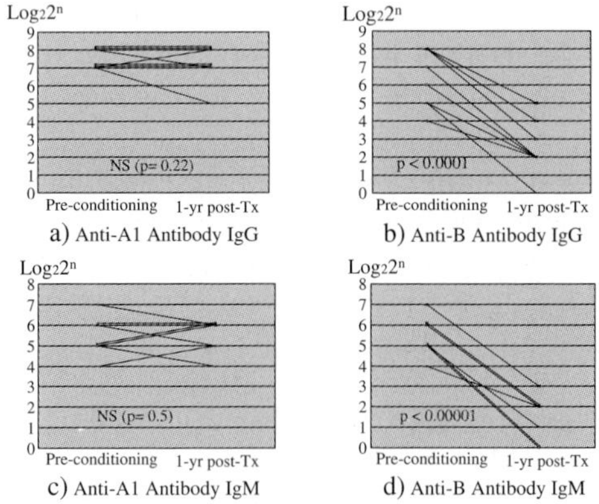

Fig. 1. Donor-specific antibody suppression in (B-to-O) (N=8).

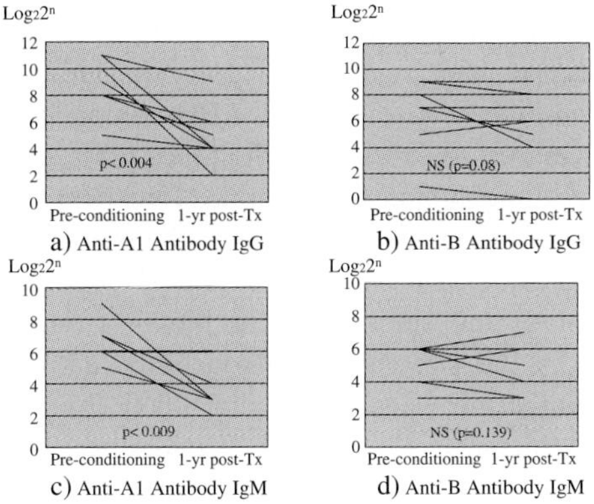

Fig. 2. Donor-specific antibody suppression in (A1-to-O) (N=7).

Intensity and pattern of staining in blood group antigens were similar under any time and conditions. There was no significant deposition of IgG, IgM and complement components with immunofluorescence in any graft specimen.

4. Discussion

B lymphocyte and plasma cell can produce both anti-A1 and anti-B antibodies in the recipients with blood group O. Antibody production must be suppressed under immunosuppression. Therefore, we compared the titers of blood group antibodies in (B-to-O) and (A1-to-O) with (O-to-O) under similar dose and kinds of immunosuppression more than 1 year post-transplantation. Only the titers of anti-donor antibodies (both of IgG and IgM) were significantly lower in (B-to-O) and (A1-to-O) than those in (O-to-O). We also studied change of the titers of blood group antibodies between pre-conditioning and 1 year post-transplantation in (B-to-O) and (A1-to-O). Only the titers of anti-donor blood group antibodies (both IgG and IgM) were significantly lower 1 year post-transplantation than those pre-conditioning although donor compatible antibodies did not differ between them. This could be explained by two theories. One is absorbance of anti-donor blood group antibodies to the blood group antigens, which were expressed in a renal allograft. Another is donor-specific suppression of anti-donor blood group antibodies. Absorbance of anti-donor antibodies seems to be unlikely because IgG, IgM and complement components were never stained properly with immunofluorescence in any biopsy specimen. West demonstrated absence of intragraft deposition of immunoglobulins and complement components in pediatric heart transplant patients [3]. Morozumi et al. also reported that immunofluorescent microscopy, revealed no significant deposition of IgG and IgM; and ordinary complements of C1q, C3 and C4 in all materials, even with severe acute humoral rejection [4]. Production of anti-donor antibodies could be specifically suppressed in long-term ABO-incompatible kidney transplant recipients. Fan et al. [5] and West [3,6] suggested that this was caused by the development of B cell tolerance. West proved that B cell tolerance was induced by elimination of donor-reactive B lymphocytes by ELISA and ELISPOT analysis [3].

Interestingly, anti-A1 antibodies persisted high titers in the recipient (A1-to-O) with delayed hyperacute rejection after removal of graft. In addition, the titers of anti-A1 antibodies maintained the high level even after ABO-compatible retransplantation under immunosuppression. In contrast, the recipient who failed graft function without removal of graft due to chronic allograft nephropathy maintained low titer (< × 32) after reintroduction to hemodialysis. Staining of blood group antigens in the protocol biopsy specimen 7 years post-transplantation demonstrated long-term existence of blood group antigens in the renal allograft. These suggested that donor-specific blood group antibodies suppression appeared to be induced by the existence of blood group antibodies. Fan et al. [5] and West [3,6] also suggested that persistence of donor blood group antigens is necessary for the process of B cell tolerance to develop. Donor-specific blood group antibody suppression appeared to be a key to promise long-term ABO-incompatible renal allograft survival.

References

[1] A. Aikawa, et al., Clinical outcome and accommodation in ABO incompatible kidney transplantation, in: J.M. Cecka, P.I. Terasaki (Eds.), Clinical Transplants 2004, UCLA Immunogenetics Center, Los Angeles, 2005, pp. 135–142.

[2] A. Aikawa, et al., Donor specific antibody suppression in ABO incompatible kidney transplantation, Transplant. Proc. 33 (2001) 395–397.

[3] L.J. West, ABO-incompatible paediatric heart transplantation, Abstract of International Conference of ABO Incompatible Transplantation, Niigata, Japan, 2005, pp. 142–143.

[4] K. Morozumi, et al., Pathologic characteristics of acute humoral rejection after ABO-incompatible kidney transplantation, Transplant. Proc. 33 (2001) 3299–3300.

[5] X. Fan, et al., Donor-specific B-cell tolerance after ABO-incompatible infant heart transplantation, Nat. Med. 10 (2004) 1227–1233 Epub.

[6] L.J. West, Targeting antibody-mediated rejection in the setting of ABO-incompatible infant heart transplantation: graft accommodation vs. B cell tolerance, Curr. Drug Targets Cardiovasc. Haematol. Disord. 5 (2005) 223–232.

International Congress Series 1292 (2006) 13–21
www.ics-elsevier.com

Severe rejection of rat intestinal grafts overexpressing human histo-blood group A/B transferase

Seiichiro Inoue [a,b], Kazunori Tahara [a,c], Jun Fujishiro [a,c], Wendy Zhou [d], Hideki Ohdan [d], Toshimasa Asahara [d], Kohei Hasnizume [c], Michio Kaneko [b], Yoji Hakamata [a], Koichi Takeuchi [e], Sadahiko Iwamoto [f], Eiji Kobayashi [a,*]

[a] *Division of Organ Replacement Research, Center for Molecular Medicine, Jichi Medical School, 3311-1 Yakushiji, Minamikawachi-machi, Kawachi-gun, Tochigi, 329-0498, Japan*
[b] *Department of Pediatric Surgery, University of Tsukuba, Japan*
[c] *Department of Pediatric Surgery, Faculty of Medicine, University of Tokyo, Japan*
[d] *Department of Surgery, University of Hiroshima, Japan*
[e] *Department of Anatomy, Jichi Medical School, Japan*
[f] *Department of Legal Medicine and Human Genetics, Jichi Medical School, Japan*

Abstract. *Background:* To test the effect of overexpressed human A/B antigens on rat immunity, we have developed transgenic (Tg) rats with human blood group A/B transferase genes in a previous report. Using these rats whose intestine expressed the A/B antigen, we tested the antigenecity of overexpressed A/B antigens in intestinal tracts. *Materials and methods:* Wild-type (MHC haplotype: $RT1^k$) and human histo-blood A or B transferase gene transgenic (A- or B-Tg) Wistar rats were used. We tested rejection reaction in heterotopic small bowel transplantation (SBT). Then, we conducted SBT and measured changes in rat anti-human blood type A antibody titers. *Results:* Small intestinal grafts from Tg to wild-type rats were severely rejected (A-Tg grafts, 19.8 ± 5.6 days; B-Tg grafts, 14.3 ± 4.6 days). Serologic study showed that rat anti-human A antibody was detected in both adult A- and B-Tg rats, but not in wild-type rats. Grafts from wild-type and Tg rats were more rapidly rejected in Tg rat recipients (7.9 ± 2.9 days). The rat anti-human A antibody titer in the Tg rat

Abbreviations: A-Transferase, α1,3-*N*-acetylgalactosamide transferase; B-Transferase, α1,3-galactosaminyl transferase; Tg, transgenic; SBT, small bowel transplantation; CSBT, cervical SBT; ELISA, enzyme-linked immunosorbent assay; OPD, *o*-phenylenediamine.

* Corresponding author. Tel.: +81 285 58 7446; fax: +81 285 44 5365.
E-mail address: eijikoba@jichi.ac.jp (E. Kobayashi).

0531-5131/ © 2006 Published by Elsevier B.V.
doi:10.1016/j.ics.2006.03.056

recipients with wild-type intestine was significantly elevated after SBT. *Conclusion:* Rat intestinal grafts overexpressing human histo-blood group A/B transferase were severely rejected, inducing humoral antibody production.

Keywords: ABO blood type antigen; Transgenic rat; Small bowel transplantation; A/B transferase

1. Introduction

ABO-mismatched organ transplantation is considered a possible solution to the donor shortage for organ transplantation. Although ABO-incompatible paring is usually contraindicated in organ transplantation, many therapeutic improvements have shown the possibility of using ABO-mismatched grafts especially in liver and renal transplantation [1,2]. Anti-A/B antibodies existing in the recipient bind to blood A/B antigens, inducing a hyperacute rejection reaction [3]. ABO-incompatible renal transplantation has been established as a therapeutic approach by overcoming the humoral barrier [4].

In the field of experimental transplantation immunology, pre-sensitized models of rat or mouse [5,6] have been established and used to mimic clinical hyperacute organ rejection using the method of pre-transplanting skin grafts. However, these were targeting the Major histocompatibility complex (MHC) and little is known about rodent A/B antigen system [7,8]. A/B antigens are oligosaccharides, not restricted to humans but are widely present in nature. We recently successfully cloned rat A/B genes and showed their equivalence to humans [8]. Using this rat model that overexpressed A/B transferase in the small intestine, we performed rat heterotopic segmental small bowel transplantation and evaluated both antigenicity and rejection.

2. Materials and method

2.1. Rat

Male wild-type Wister rats (MHC haplotype: $RT1^k$) purchased from CLEA Japan (Tokyo, Japan), and human blood type A-/B-transferase gene transgenic Wistar rats (A-/B-Tg rat), originally developed by us [8] were used in these experiments. All experiments of this study were performed in accordance with the Jichi Medical School Guide for Laboratory Animals.

2.2. Establishment of human A- and B-transferase Tg rats

Establishment of Human A-/B-transferase Tg rats was previously reported [8]. Briefly, to establish A-/B-transferase Tg rats, human blood type A/B transferase cDNAs were used. Human A-transferase cDNA isoform, which was kindly provided by Dr. Hakomori [8,9], includes intron 6 of the human ABO gene (FY-66-1); and human B-transferase cDNA generated by replacement of the *Sac*II/*Sal*I fragment of FY-66-1 with that of B-transferase gene exon 7 of the human ABO gene. Each cDNA was inserted to the downstream of the chicken β-actin promoter of the pCAGGS vector and was injected into Wistar rat nuclei. Then the microinjected fertilized eggs were transferred to pseudopregnant rats. Stable lines of Tg rats were generated by breeding the founders with detecting of tail genomic DNA and total RNA by PCR and RT–PCR.

A and B antigen expression in A-, B-Tg and wild Wistar rats was confirmed by immunohistochemical staining. A quantitative evaluation of ABH antigen expression in the small intestine was performed by Western blot analysis.

The immunohistochemical staining of A-, B-Tg and wild Wistar rat small intestine was also performed previously [8]. Small intestines from A-/B-Tg and wild Wistar rats were stained with anti-A or anti-B antibodies, then with biotin-labeled anti-mouse goat antibody, and finally with Texas Red-labeled avidin. Nuclei counterstaining was performed using 4′,6-diamino-2-phenylindole. Because human histo-blood type A or B antigens were well expressed in these small bowels, we used this organ to perform the transplantation experiments in this report.

2.3. Detection of anti-human blood type A antibody in A- or B-Tg rats

Although the detection of serum anti-human blood type A/B antibodies are very important for the ABO-mismatched organ transplantation, the methods of detecting them in rodents have not been established. Zhou and Ohdan et al. established and reported the novel method of measuring the mouse serum anti-human A antibody (IgM and IgG) using of synthetic A determinant-BSA by the enzyme-linked immunosorbent assay (ELISA) method [7]. We applied this method to measure the rat anti-human A antibody. Briefly, 96-well flat-bottomed microplates were coated with 5 μl/ml of goat anti-human Ig (Southern Biotechnology Associates, Birmingham, AL), 5 μg/ml of synthetic A determinant-BSA (GalNAcα1–3Fucα$_1$αGal-BSA) (Dextra, Reading, UK) or 5 μg/ml of control BSA. Diluted serum samples were incubated in the microplates and bound antibodies were detected using horseradish peroxidase-conjugated goat anti-human immunoglobulin specific antibodies (KOL, Guilford, UK). Color development was achieved using 0.1 mg/ml *o*-phenylenediamine (OPD) (Sigma Chemical Co., St Louis, MO) in a substrate buffer. The color reaction was stopped by adding 3 M H_2SO_4 and absorption values at 492 nm were obtained with micro-plate reader. Rat anti-human A-specific antibodies levels were determined by subtraction of the absorbance of wells coated with control BSA from the absorbance of wells coated with A-conjugated BSA. Human purified IgG (Zymed. S. San Francisco, CA) and IgM (ICN Biomedicals, Aurora, OH) were used as standard controls.

2.4. Cervical small bowel transplantation (CSBT) in rats

To test the immunological reaction after organ transplantation, we performed heterotopic small bowel transplantation [10]. Briefly, after a transverse incision on the donor abdomen, the colonic vessels were ligated and dissected. The distal end of the intestine graft was first cut, and then proximal end was cut 15 cm from the anal end. The portal vein was gently separated from the pancreas. The aorta was ligated above the origin of the superior mesenteric artery and mobilized. After injection of 200 U of heparin, the intestinal lumen was flushed with 20 ml saline to remove the contents. The aorta containing the superior mesenteric artery was dissected. A diagonal cut was made at the intersection of the portal vein and the splenic vein, and the small bowel and its vascular supply were removed. Under ether anesthesia, a neck skin incision was made. The common carotid artery and jugular vein were dissected free and bundled with microclips. The cuffs were attached to the vessels using a 20-G (for vein) and 16-G (for artery) Teflon tube (Surflo, Terumo Co., Ltd., Tokyo, Japan). The portal vein and the aorta of the graft were connected to the recipient jugular vein and carotid artery, respectively. The proximal and distal ends of the short grafts were exteriorized as stomas. The recipient rats were allowed free access to water and foods. The rats were weighed two to three times per week. The stoma were observed daily, and the day when the stoma closed and remained dry was defined as the day of graft rejection.

2.5. Histopathologic evaluation

To investigate the graft histologically, biopsies were taken from the stoma at 1, 2, and 3 weeks after transplantation. The biopsy specimens were fixed with 10% paraformaldehyde and stained with hematoxylin and eosin.

3. Experimental protocol

3.1. Experiment I. Antigenicity of human histo-blood A- or B-antigen overexpression in the intestinal graft

To evaluate the antigenicity of human A- or B-overexpression in A- or B-Tg rats, we performed CSBT using A- or B-Tg rat small intestinal graft as the donor and wild-type rats as the recipients. The control consisted of wild-type rat small intestine transplanted to wild-type recipients.

3.2. Experiment II. Production of rat anti-human A antibody in A- or B-Tg rats

Serum rat anti-human A antibody level in wild-type and A- or B-Tg rats was measured as described above. Tail vein blood was obtained at 4, 6, 8 and 10 weeks from A- and B-Tg rats, and from 6- and 8-week-old wild Wistar rats and assayed by ELISA for the presence of rat anti-human A antibody.

Next, to investigate the effect of rat anti-human A antibody on the rejection of an intestinal graft, we performed CSBT using A- and B-Tg rats as the recipients, since human anti-A antibody was detected in A- and B-Tg serum but not in wild-type serum. We also tested the production of rat anti-human A antibody in A- and B-Tg rats when they were sensitized with blood type A antigen. Rat serum anti-human A antibody levels before and after CSBT were assayed by ELISA.

4. Results

4.1. Expression of human blood type ABH antigen in A-, B-Tg rats and wild Wistar rats

The basic genomic background and details of gene expression regarding human histo-blood group ABH antigens in the wild-type and A- or B-Tg rats have been previously reported [8]. Wild-type rats expressed A-antigen on the salivary gland, mucosal crypts, intestinal mucous and epithelium of the urinary bladder, and weakly on stomach epithelium. Enhanced expression of A-antigen by the human histo-blood A-transferase transgene was observed in the brain plexus, type II lung epithelium, pancreas, and the epidermis. Anti-B antigen staining was not observed in wild-type or A-Tg rats, whereas weak expression of rat B-transferase mRNA was ubiquitous. B-antigens were expressed in B-Tg rat in organs identical to that for A-Tg rats. The salivary glands, stomach,

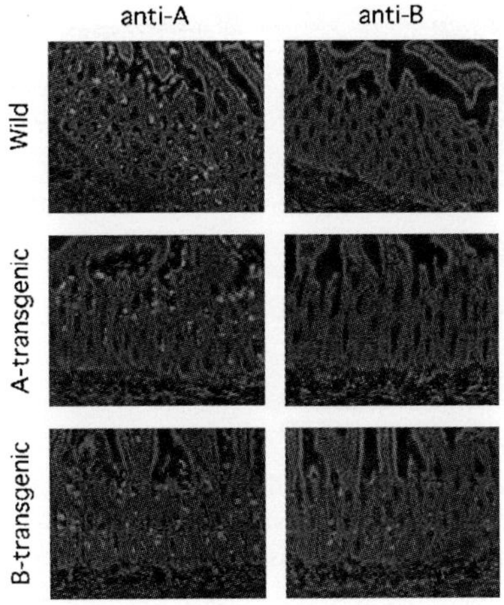

Fig. 1. Immunohistochemical staining of A- or B-antigen in wild-type, A- and B-Tg rat small intestine. A- or B-antigens expressed in the small intestine are shown in red, and nuclei are shown in blue. In the wild-type small intestine, A-antigen was expressed but not B-antigen. Overexpression of A-antigen was observed in A-Tg small intestine, although expression of B-antigen was not detected. In the B-Tg small intestine, expression of both A and B antigens was detected. (For interpretation of the references to colour in this figure legend, the reader is referred to the web version of this article.)

intestine, and bladder of B-Tg rats were positive for anti-A antibody. Photos of immunohistological staining of small intestines from wild Wistar and A- or B-Tg rats are shown in Fig. 1.

4.2. Rejection reaction to overexpressed human histo-blood A- or B-blood type antigens

Graft survival after CSBT in wild-type recipient is shown in Table 1. Small intestinal grafts from A-Tg rats were rejected from 12 to 25 days after transplantation (mean ± S.D. = 19.8 ± 5.6 days), and grafts from B-Tg rats were rejected from 9 to 20 days after transplantation (14.3 ± 4.6 days), whereas grafts from wild-type rats survived more than 30 days after transplantation.

Representative histopathologic stains at 2 weeks after transplantation are shown in Fig. 2a,b,c. In A-Tg to wild-type rats, mononuclear cell infiltration into the villi was observed at 1 week after transplantation. By 2 weeks after transplantation, destruction of the mucosal

Table 1
Graft survival after CSBT using A- and B-Tg rats

Donor	Recipient	*N*	Graft survival (days)	Mean ± S.D.
Wild	Wild	5	>30, >30, >30, >30, >30	>30
A-Tg	Wild	4	12, 20, 22, 25	19.8 ± 5.6
B-Tg	Wild	4	9, 13, 15, 20	14.3 ± 4.6
Wild	A-Tg	4	5, 6, 7, 8	6.5 ± 1.3
Wild	B-Tg	4	6, 8, 8, 8	7.5 ± 1.0
B-Tg	A-Tg	4	4, 8, 10, 15	9.3 ± 4.6
A-Tg	B-Tg	4	5, 6, 11, 12	8.5 ± 3.5

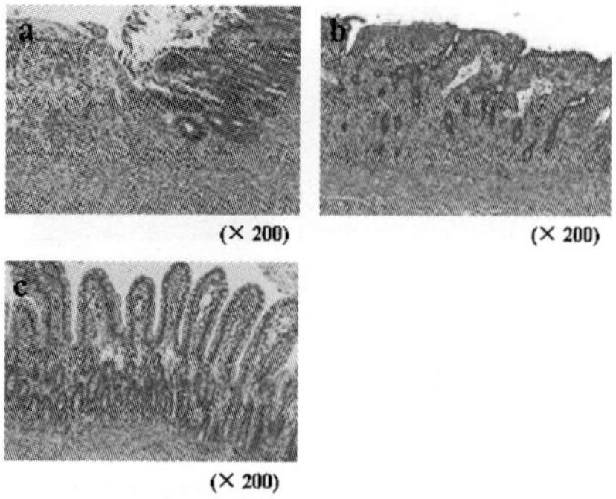

Fig. 2. Microscopic appearance of transplanted small intestinal grafts at 14 days after CSBT using wild-type recipients (hematoxylin and eosin staining). (a) Small intestinal graft from A-Tg rats was transplanted to wild type recipients. Massive cell infiltration with patchy necrosis of the intestinal mucosa was observed in the graft from an A-Tg rat. Small intestinal villi were partially observed (magnification ×200). (b) Graft from B-Tg rat was used. Complete structural destruction of small intestinal mucosa with massive cell infiltration was seen (magnification ×200). (c) Wild-type intestine was used as a control. Structure of wild-type intestine was almost normal (magnification ×200).

structure was partially observed, but normal intestinal wall structure with cell infiltrations was also observed in grafts at 3 weeks after transplantation. B-Tg grafts were rejected more severely than A-Tg grafts. At 2 weeks after transplantation, hemorrhagic necrosis was observed in the grafted intestinal wall, and by 3 weeks after transplantation, the intestinal wall structure was completely destroyed. In controls, normal graft intestinal wall structure was observed at 3 weeks after transplantation.

4.3. Rat anti-human blood type A-antibody production by A- and B-Tg rats

In the wild-type Wistar rats that did not perform any transplantation, only very limited levels of rat anti-human A specific antibodies were detected ($OD=0.077 \pm 0.007$, $n=6$). However, rat anti-human A antibody was detected in A- and B-Tg rats (Fig. 3a,c). As shown in Fig. 3a, rat anti-human A antibody was constantly produced in 4- to 10-week-old A-Tg rats. On the other hand, young (4- to 6-week-old) B-Tg rats produced more rat anti-human A antibody than A-Tg rats; however, after 8 weeks, B-Tg rats produced comparable levels with A-Tg rats as shown in Fig. 3c.

4.4. Sensitization by wild-type small intestines that express A-antigen in A- and B-Tg rats

Serum rat anti-human A antibody levels before and after heterotopic small bowel transplantation in A- and B-Tg rat recipients are shown in Fig. 3b,d. In both groups, two of four recipients were sensitized with wild-type rat small intestinal grafts, and produced rat anti-human A antibody. In the A-Tg rats group, the rat anti-human A antibody level did not increase in one recipient, and in another recipient, the OD value decreased to less than 0 after control absorbance subtraction, which was indicative of high levels of another nonspecific antibody. In B-Tg rats, rat anti-human A antibodies did not increase.

Graft survival and histologic staining of small intestine grafts at 2 weeks after SBT with recipient A- and B-Tg rats are shown in Table 1 and Fig. 4. Compared with the groups with wild-type recipient rats (Table 1 and Fig. 2) these grafts were more rapidly and more

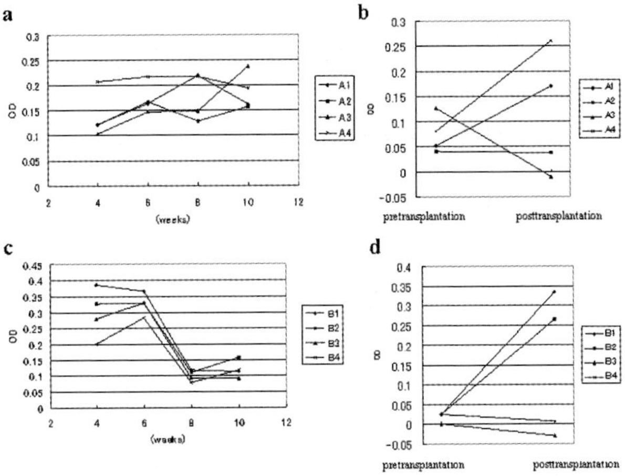

Fig. 3. Change in human blood anti-A antibody titers before and after CSBT. Rat anti-human A antibodies were detected in A-Tg (a) and B-Tg (c) serum, but not in wild-type rats. Serum human anti-A antibody titers were elevated in 50% of A-Tg (b) and B-Tg (d) recipients after sensitization with wild-type small intestine.

severely rejected by A- and B-Tg recipients. At 2 weeks after SBT, the grafts were severely rejected and small intestinal structures such as the mucosa, submucosal layer and muscular layer were completely destroyed with severe cell infiltration.

5. Discussion

Antibody-mediated (humoral) rejection is the most important factor in ABO-mismatched organ transplantation. Since binding antibody to the A/B antigen expressed in the graft is the initial step of a hyperacute rejection in ABO-mismatch transplantation, many reports indicate that ABO-incompatible liver and renal grafts can be protected after

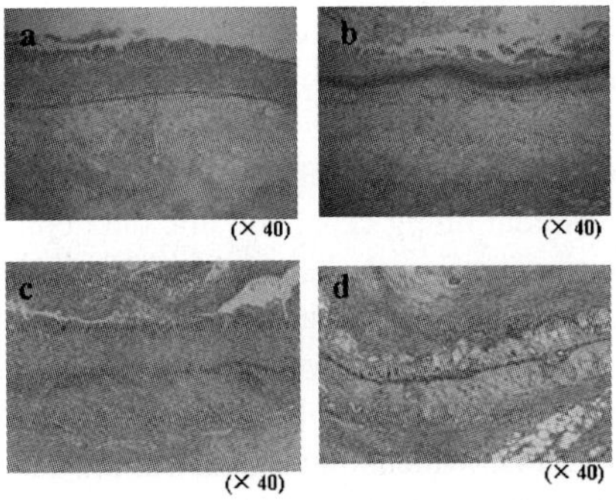

Fig. 4. Microscopic appearance of transplanted small intestinal grafts at 14 days after CSBT using A- or B-Tg rat as recipients (hematoxylin and eosin staining). (a) Wild-type intestine was transplanted to A-Tg rat. (b) Wild-type intestine was transplanted to B-Tg rat. Massive cell infiltration into the mucosa, submucosal and smooth muscle layer and destruction of mucosa structure were observed in both grafts (magnification ×40). (c) Small intestinal graft from A-Tg rat was transplanted to B-Tg recipient. (d) Graft from B-Tg rat was transplanted to A-Tg recipient. Both grafts showed complete destruction of the intestinal wall (hemorrhagic necrosis) (magnification ×40).

transplantation by removing A or B antibody prior to, at the time of, and after transplantation [2,11–15]. Many therapeutic modalities for removing antibodies or suppressing the production of antibody have been reported including splenectomy and/or anti-metabolic immunosuppressants [11,12,16,17].

The expression of A/B antigens and the production of antibody are critical factors for an ABO-mismatch transplantation model. In our previous study, we successfully developed A- or B-transferase Tg rats that overexpressed the human A or B blood antigen [8]. In this study, we demonstrate that these overexpressed antigens located in the small intestine have antigenicity and function as antigens. Moreover, we also demonstrated that A- and B-Tg rats have the ability to produce rat anti-human blood type A antibody, although the mechanism is unclear. Since blood type A antigens were originally expressed in the intestine of wild Wistar rats, Tg rats could be sensitized.

However, several points are unclear and the mechanisms are unknown in this process. Because the wild Wistar rat is an out-bred strain, small intestinal grafts were rejected in wild-type recipients after more than 30 days after transplantation. However, small intestinal grafts from wild-type rats were rapidly rejected in A- or B-Tg recipients, although wild Wistar rats had A antigen expression [8]. Yet, tolerance against A antigens was not induced in A- and B-Tg rats. Moreover, A- and B-Tg rats sensitized by wild-type rat small intestine had elevated A antibody after CSBT. The mechanisms of these phenomena are still unclear and further investigations are warranted.

In order to establish a rat model that completely mimics clinical ABO-mismatch organ transplantation, further refinements may be needed. For example, grafts were rejected about 7 to 14 days after transplantation in this study. However, humoral rejections can appear immediately after organ transplantation. To mimic this phenomenon, pre-sensitization using several skin transplantations and elevation of the rat anti-human A antibody level before organ transplantation may be possible and effective. Moreover, A and B antigens are not expressed in the liver and kidney in Tg rats. The immunodominant parts of the A/B antigens bind to the core chain H antigen. The A or B antigen is converted from the H antigen by A or B transferase [1,18,19]. Overexpressed A or B antigens are synthesized from H antigen that existed in the wild-type rats, because only the A or B transferase gene was transferred to the Tg rats. In the human kidney, human anti A/B antigens are primarily expressed in the vascular endothelium, the glomeruli, the interstitium, and the tubules [1]. These antigens are expressed on the hepatic artery, portal vein, capillaries, sinusoidal lining cells, and bile duct epithelium in human liver [1]. Yet, expression of these antigens was not observed in Tg rats [8]. To overcome this issue, additional gene transfer encoding human H-antigen targeting the expression of H antigen to these organs or structures may be effective, and we are planning such experiments.

In conclusion, we demonstrated that human histo-blood A/B transferase gene transgenic rats' intestinal grafts, which overexpressed with human A/B antigen, were severely and rapidly rejected, and that overexpressed A/B antigens can act as antigens in an ABO-mismatched organ transplantation model. Human A-/B-transferase gene transgenic rats have the ability to produce circulating rat anti-human A antibody. This antibody can accelerate the rejection against A antigens that were expressed on Tg and wild Wistar rat small intestinal grafts. Additional investigations may enable us to refine an ABO-mismatch organ transplantation model in rats.

Acknowledgments

This work is supported by a grant from the Research on Health Sciences focusing on Drug Innovation to E.K.

References

[1] L. Rydberg, ABO-incompatibility in solid organ transplantation, Transfus. Med. 11 (2001) 325–342.
[2] H. Toma, K. Tanabe, T. Tokumoto, Long-term outcome of ABO-incompatible renal transplantation, Urol. Clin. North Am. 28 (2001) 769–780.
[3] R.L. Jenkins, et al., ABO mismatch and liver transplantation, Transplant. Proc. 19 (1987) 4580–4585.
[4] G.P. Alexandre, et al., Present experiences in a series of 26 ABO-incompatible living donor renal allografts, Transplant. Proc. 19 (1987) 4538–4542.
[5] R.D. Guttmann, Genetics of acute rejection of rat cardiac allografts and a model of hyperacute rejection, Transplantation 17 (1974) 383–386.
[6] F. Fu, et al., Prevention and restoration of second-set liver allograft rejection in presensitized mice: the role of "passenger" leukocytes, donor major histocompatibility complex antigens, and host cytotoxic effector mechanisms, Transplantation 67 (1999) 444–450.
[7] W. Zhou, et al., NOD/SCID mice engrafted with human peripheral blood lymphocytes can be a model for investigating B cells responding to blood group A carbohydrate determinant, Transplant. Immunol. 12 (2003) 9–18.
[8] S. Iwamoto, et al., Rat encodes the paralogous gene equivalent of the human histo-blood group ABO gene. Association with antigen expression by overexpression of human ABO transferase, J. Biol. Chem. 277 (2002) 46463–46469.
[9] F. Yamamoto, P.D. McNeill, S. Hakomori, Genomic organization of human histo-blood group ABO genes, Glycobiology 5 (1995) 51–58.
[10] S. Inoue, et al., Impact of graft length on surgical damage after intestinal transplantation in rats, Transplant. Immunol. 11 (2003) 207–214.
[11] T. Sawada, S. Fuchinoue, S. Teraoka, Successful A1-to-O ABO-incompatible kidney transplantation after a preconditioning regimen consisting of anti-CD20 monoclonal antibody infusions, splenectomy, and double-filtration plasmapheresis, Transplantation 74 (2002) 1207–1210.
[12] D.W. Hanto, et al., ABO-incompatible liver transplantation with no immunological graft losses using total plasma exchange, splenectomy, and quadruple immunosuppression: evidence for accommodation, Liver Transplant. 9 (2003) 22–30.
[13] W.I. Bensinger, et al., Immunoadsorption for removal of A and B blood-group antibodies, N. Engl. J. Med. 304 (1981) 160–162.
[14] T. Yandza, et al., Outcome of ABO-incompatible liver transplantation in children with no specific alloantibodies at the time of transplantation, Transplantation 58 (1994) 46–50.
[15] K. Ota, et al., Multicentre trial of ABO-incompatible kidney transplantation. Japanese Biosynsorb ABO-incompatible kidney transplant study group, Transpl. Int. 5 (Suppl. 1) (1992) S40–S43.
[16] M. Tanabe, et al., Intraportal infusion therapy as a novel approach to adult ABO-incompatible liver transplantation, Transplantation 73 (2002) 1959–1961.
[17] H. Sekido, et al., Successful adult ABO-incompatible liver transplantation: therapeutic strategy for thrombotic microangiopathy is the key to success, Transplantation 75 (2003) 1605–1607.
[18] W.M. Watkins, The ABO blood group system: historical background, Transfus. Med. 11 (2001) 243–265.
[19] F. Yamamoto, et al., Molecular genetic basis of the histo-blood group ABO system, Nature 345 (1990) 229–233.

Pathology

International Congress Series 1292 (2006) 25–31

ELSEVIER

www.ics-elsevier.com

Correlation of conventional histology, clinical outcomes, and C4d immunostaining in ABO-incompatible liver transplantation

Hironori Haga [a,b,*], Hiromi Sakashita [b], Mei-Chin Wen [c], Aya Miyagawa-Hayashino [b], Hiroto Egawa [d], Toshiaki Manabe [b]

[a] *Organ Transplant Unit, Kyoto University Hospital, Kyoto, Japan*
[b] *Laboratory of Diagnostic Pathology, Kyoto University Hospital, Japan*
[c] *Department of Pathology, Taichung Veterans General Hospital, Taichung, Taiwan*
[d] *Transplantation Immunology, Kyoto University Hospital, Kyoto, Japan*

Abstract. In ABO blood type-incompatible liver transplantation (ABO-I LT), acute humoral rejection triggered by antibodies against donor-type isoagglutinins is the most serious form of rejection and often associated with graft loss. Typical histology of humoral rejection is recognized by biopsies taken at the onset of elevation of alloantibody titers; such biopsies reveal marked portal edema with or without hemorrhagic necrosis. Edema disappears several days after the onset of humoral rejection, and follow-up biopsies reveal relatively nonspecific findings such as hepatocyte necrosis or cholangitis-like portal fibrosis. In our series enrolled between 1995 and 2004, hemorrhagic portal edema was recognized in 17 of 114 (15%) patients who underwent primary ABO-I LT. All 17 patients showed elevation of anti-donor A/B IgM antibody titers (1:64 or higher), and 6-month graft survival was 59%. Deposition of C4d in portal stroma was demonstrated in 11 of 12 (92%) patients with hemorrhagic portal edema and some patients with other histology showing high postoperative alloantibody titers. Although more study is needed, these results suggest that C4d immunostaining can be a useful marker to demonstrate humoral rejection in ABO-I LT. © 2006 Published by Elsevier B.V.

Keywords: Humoral rejection; Antibody-mediated rejection; Periportal edema and necrosis; Rejection activity index; C4d

* Corresponding author. Laboratory of Diagnostic Pathology, Kyoto University Hospital, 54 Kawahara-cho Shogoin, Sakyo-ku, Kyoto 606-8507, Japan. Tel.: +81 75 751 3488; fax: +81 75 751 3499.

E-mail address: haga@kuhp.kyoto-u.ac.jp (H. Haga).

0531-5131/ © 2006 Published by Elsevier B.V.
doi:10.1016/j.ics.2006.03.068

1. Introduction

Humoral, or antibody-mediated, rejection is believed as a relatively uncommon form of allograft injury in liver transplantation. Some unusual pattern of graft failure may be associated with humoral rejection [1,2]. It is of note, however, that some antibody-mediated rejection may be overlooked because of lack of appropriate monitoring and histological assessment.

Histological assessment is often problematic because of difficulty of demonstrating anti-donor antibody and subsequent complement activation in the graft [3]. Histological findings of humoral rejection will depend on the timing of biopsy and type of alloantibodies and preconditioning against anti-humoral rejection.

In (emergent) ABO blood type-incompatible liver transplantation (ABO-I LT) some earlier reports emphasized changes in sinusoids such as congestion, neutrophilic infiltration, and deposits of immunoglobulins [3,4]. Although these lobular changes are conspicuous, it is unlikely that sinusoids are primary targets of ABO-incompatible humoral rejection since ABH histo-blood group antigens are weakly expressed in sinusoids and hepatocytes. Strong expression of ABO blood-type antigens is usually seen in capillaries in the portal tracts [5]. In our series of planned ABO-I LT with preoperative plasmapheresis periportal edema and necrosis seen at the elevation of alloantibody titers were associated with severe graft damage [6]. More recent reports from other groups showed that portal hemorrhage and edema without significant necrosis could be successfully treated by anti-humoral rejection therapy [7,8]. In animal models of humoral rejection, periportal changes could be seen as early as several hours after revascularization [9]. In recent human ABO-I LT, preoperative antibody depletion by plasmapheresis is performed and humoral rejection does not occur in hyperacute fashion; portal edema is usually seen 5–6 days after transplantation with re-elevation of anti-donor antibody titer [6–8]. We have not experienced ABO-incompatible humoral rejection that started > 3 weeks posttransplantation. Follow-up biopsies often reveal either massive necrosis (severe form) or cholangitis (milder form) and severe irreversible graft damage is common after humoral rejection [3,4,6].

In this paper, we present a short review of clinicopathological findings of our ABO-I LT series including the results of C4d immunostaining. C4d is a useful marker of antibody-mediated rejection in kidney and heart transplantation, but its significance in liver transplantation has been poorly understood.

2. Methods

2.1. Patient selection

Between January 1995 and December 2004, 114 patients (62 children and 52 adults) received primary ABO-incompatible living donor liver transplantation. For all patients, data of postoperative anti-donor A/B antibody titers were available. Among pediatric patients, 45 were aged < 3 years. Patients underwent preoperative plasmapheresis or blood exchange to reduce anti-donor blood group A/B antibody (IgM and IgG) titers to 1:8 or lower. Recent adult patients underwent continuous prostaglandin E1 infusion via intraarterial or intravenous catheter for 2–3 weeks posttransplantation [10]. Splenectomy or administration of preoperative rituximab was also performed in adult patients.

Postoperative plasmapheresis was performed when severe humoral rejection was clinically or histologically suggested. As of September 2005, the clinical follow-up period for these patients ranged from 0.4 to 126 (median 30) months. Among them, 58 patients (26 adults and 32 children, 21 aged < 3 years) underwent liver biopsy within the first 3 postoperative weeks. Since we do not perform protocol biopsy for humoral rejection, all biopsies were related to graft dysfunction.

2.2. Histological assessment

Histological humoral rejection was suspected when portal edema with or without hemorrhagic necrosis was associated with elevation of anti-donor A/B IgM antibody titers (1:64 or more). In each case of acute cellular rejection and humoral rejection, portal inflammation, bile duct damage, and venular endothelialitis were separately evaluated with rejection activity index (RAI) of Banff criteria [11]. To apply RAI to humoral rejection, we regarded any leukocyte infiltration as portal inflammation and gave a score of 3 on periportal coagulative necrosis as part of portal inflammation.

2.3. Immunohistochemistry

Polyclonal antibody against C4d complement (BI-RC4D; Biomedica, Austria, 1:50) was used for immunostaining by automated immunostainer (BENCHMARK®XT, Ventana, USA). For antigen retrieval, deparaffinized and rehydrated sections were treated with protease I (Ventana, 0.5 units/mL) at 37 °C for 20 min. Lymph nodes with follicular hyperplasia were used as positive controls for C4d staining. Time-zero allograft biopsies were used as negative control.

2.4. Statistics

Statistical significance of differences among groups was assessed by Fisher's exact test. Laboratory data was analyzed by Mann–Whitney's *U*-test.

3. Results

3.1. Histology and clinical outcomes

Fifty-six of 114 (49%) patients did not undergo biopsy in the first 3 postoperative weeks, and their 6-month graft survival was 84% (Table 1).

Table 1
Histology of first postoperative biopsies of 114 primary ABO-I LT in Kyoto University between January 1995 and December 2004

Histology[a]	Not available ($n=56$)	ACR/lobular inflammation ($n=20$)	Cholangitis/ centrilobular necrosis ($n=21$)	Humoral rejection ($n=17$)
Age < 3 years	43%	75%	28%	0%
High alloantibody IgM titer (1:64 or more)	32%	35%	52%	100%
Six-month graft survival	84%	80%	71%	59%
Stromal C4d	3/7 (43%)	1/9 (11%)	6/17 (35%)	11/12 (91%)

[a] First biopsies taken within the first 3 postoperative weeks.

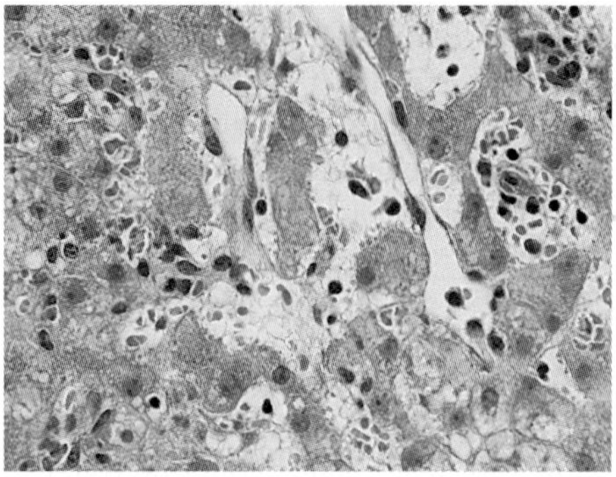

Fig. 1. Periportal edema in ABO-incompatible humoral rejection (postoperative day 7). Portal edema extended into periportal areas, and there was detachment of sinusoidal cells from hepatocytes. Fragmentation of red blood cells was present but these changes were subtle in routine light microscopy. The patient died of massive necrosis of hepatocytes. (For interpretation of the references to colour in this figure legend, the reader is referred to the web version of this article.)

A total of 20 (18%) patients whose first biopsy showed simple acute cellular rejection or mild lobular inflammation also showed > 80% of 6-month graft survival rate. Three quarters of them were aged < 3 years, and high postoperative titer was seen in 35% of patients.

Cholangitis/hepatocanalicular cholestasis or centrilobular necrosis was seen in 21 (18%) patients. These patients tended to be older than the acute rejection or lobular inflammation group, and postoperative high-titer was seen in about half of the patients.

Humoral rejection characterized by portal edema was seen in 17 (15%) patients (Fig. 1). Periportal edema was seen only in patients aged > 3 years and all of the patients showed high postoperative anti-donor antibody titer. Their prognoses were the worst among groups.

In patients with portal edema graft failure tended to be associated with anti-A antibody, delay of biopsy, high transaminase and serum bilirubin, and very high postoperative alloantibody titers (Table 2). Higher RAI was significantly associated with graft failure, while patients who recovered showed minimal inflammation or necrosis.

3.2. *C4d immunostaining.*

We were able to perform C4d immunostaining only in 38 recent ABO-incompatible cases (Table 3).

Table 2
Patients with humoral rejection characterized by portal edema

Results	Graft failure (n = 11)	Recovery (n = 6)	P-value
Anti-A/anti-B	8:4	2:5	0.12
POD	9.2 ± 4.3	6.5 ± 1.4	0.2
ALT (IU/L)	429 ± 460	290 ± 100	0.52
T-Bil (mg/dL)	15.7 ± 11.3	7.3 ± 3.3	0.1
Median peak IgM titer	1:2048	1:512	–
Rejection activity index	4.9 ± 2.0	2.3 ± 1.4	0.02
Portal stromal C4d	6/7 (86%)	5/5 (100%)	0.6

POD, postoperative day.

Table 3
C4d immunoreactivity in biopsies taken within first 3 postoperative weeks

Staining pattern	C4d immunostaining		*P*-value
	Diffuse stromal ± endothelial staining	Endothelial only/negative	
No. of patients	18	20	–
POD at biopsy	10.1 ± 4.9	14.5 ± 4.6	0.01
Age < 3 years	3 (17%)	7 (35%)	0.18
High IgM titer (1:64 or more)	16 (89%)	9 (45%)	0.005
Portal edema	11 (61%)	1 (5%)	< 0.0002
Six-month survival	10 (56%)	17 (85%)	0.05

We interpreted portal stromal staining as specific staining pattern for humoral rejection. Biopsies containing > 50% stromal-positive portal tracts were evaluated as positive (Fig. 2, left). Linear endothelial staining in portal blood vessels was commonly seen in stromal-positive cases (Fig. 2, right). Faint or endothelial-only staining was not associated with ominous histology or poor prognosis and we interpreted these findings as indeterminate or not diagnostic for humoral rejection. Extra liver connective tissue or nerve fibers sometimes showed diffuse staining even in normal nontransplanted livers, and we interpreted such staining as nonspecific.

Eighteen of 38 (47%) cases were classified as C4d positive, 10 (26%) as indeterminate, and 10 (26%) as negative. Early biopsies tended to be associated with C4d stromal staining. It is of note that C4d positivity was seen in 3 patients aged < 3 years. Their histology included acute rejection, necrosis, and cholangitis, respectively, and the 2 patients without cholangitis recovered. All patients with C4d positivity were clinically suspected of humoral rejection. Although 2 of 18 patients did not show high postoperative IgM antibody titers, they were associated with high IgG titer (1:256) and T-cell crossmatch positivity, respectively. C4d stromal staining was also associated with poorer graft survival (56% vs. 85%; $P = 0.05$), although C4d-negative cases included 2 patients who developed chronic cholangitis and 1 patient with histological humoral rejection (periportal edema and necrosis).

4. Discussion

Appropriate preconditioning to prevent humoral rejection is key to successful adult-to-adult ABO-I LT [10,12]. Postoperative monitoring of anti-donor A/B antibody titers and

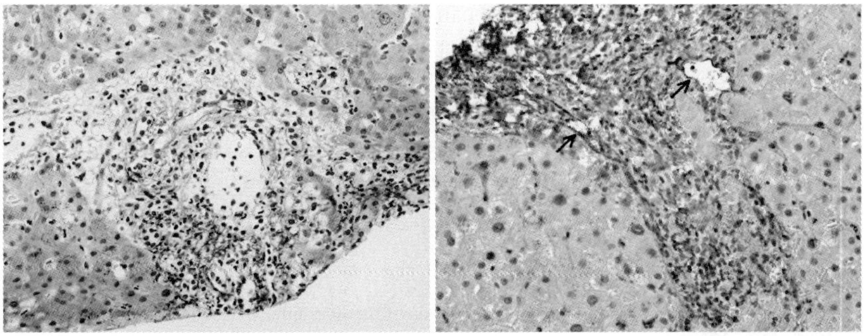

Fig. 2. (Left) Portal stromal C4d staining in humoral rejection. Periportal areas and some capillaries were positive for C4d, but the portal vein was negative. (Right) Endothelial staining in portal vein or venules (arrows).

liver enzymes usually provides enough information for diagnosis of ABO-incompatible humoral rejection. Considering these observations and the increased risk of hemorrhage after ABO-I LT, protocol biopsy may not be indicated. However, biopsy is still required in cases of humoral rejection to confirm typical histology and to evaluate severity of the disease. Early recognition of rejection is useful to evaluate typical histology of humoral rejection. In ABO-I LT, we could emphasize portal edema with or without hemorrhage as a histological feature of early humoral rejection. Rapid progression of the process seemed to efface typical periportal changes within a few days after the onset of humoral rejection [4]. Intensive treatment is required for portal edema, while anti-humoral rejection therapy after disappearance of edema and after decrease of alloantibody titers may be too late to treat.

In this report, we performed retrospective C4d immunostaining to evaluate biopsies taken after ABO-I LT. Portal stromal C4d staining, not endothelial staining only, was well correlated with portal edema, high postoperative alloantibody titer, and poor patient survival. This staining pattern was different to that in other solid organ transplantation where endothelial staining is diagnostic for humoral rejection. In ABO-I LT of our series, C4d staining restricted to the endothelium did not seem related to humoral rejection. Methods for antigen retrieval might be related to the difference of staining pattern. Or, the staining pattern in ABO-I LT may suggest that overflow of complement activation outside capillaries may be necessary to destruct blood supply of the portal tract and to cause severe liver damage. At least C4d staining pattern in humoral rejection seems associated with extensive C4d deposition in liver allograft. Clinicopathological correlation suggests that cholangitis or centrilobular necrosis showing stromal C4d deposition would be the results of humoral rejection.

Since there were some C4d-negative intrahepatic biliary dilatation cases and a C4d-negative humoral rejection case, false-negative C4d immunostaining should also be considered in some minority cases.

As a next step, incorporation of C4d into routine histological diagnosis of liver allograft biopsies will be necessary to evaluate its value other than as a marker of ABO-incompatible humoral rejection.

5. Conclusion

Portal edema was associated with elevation of postoperative alloantibody titer, C4d stromal staining, and poor prognosis and can be regarded as a useful histological feature of early-phase ABO-incompatible humoral rejection. Some cases of cholangitis and lobular necrosis may also be regarded as results of humoral rejection if they are associated with antibody titer elevation and C4d immunostaining. Since this was a retrospective study and limited numbers of specimens were available for C4d stain, further study is necessary to elucidate the significance and immunostaining pattern of C4d.

References

[1] S.G. Hubscher, et al., Massive haemorrhagic necrosis of the liver after liver transplantation, J. Clin. Pathol. 42 (1989) 360–370.

[2] M.A. Memon, et al., Seventh Day Syndrome—acute hepatocyte apoptosis associated with a unique syndrome of graft loss following liver transplantation, Liver 21 (2001) 13–17.

[3] A.J. Demetris, et al., Antibody-mediated rejection of human orthotopic liver allografts. A study of liver transplantation across ABO blood group barriers, Am. J. Pathol. 132 (1988) 489–502.
[4] J. Gugenheim, et al., Liver transplantation across ABO blood group barriers, Lancet 336 (1990) 519–523.
[5] Y. Tanaka, et al., Intragraft expression of recipient-type ABO blood group antigens: long-term follow-up and histological features after liver transplantation, Liver Transplant. 11 (2005) 547–554.
[6] H. Haga, et al., Periportal edema and necrosis as diagnostic histological features of early humoral rejection in ABO-incompatible liver transplantation, Liver Transplant. 10 (2004) 16–27.
[7] M. Usuda, et al., Successful use of anti-CD20 monoclonal antibody (rituximab) for ABO-incompatible living-related liver transplantation, Transplantation 79 (2005) 12–16.
[8] D. Morioka, et al., Antibody-mediated rejection after adult ABO-incompatible liver transplantation remedied by gamma-globulin bolus infusion combined with plasmapheresis, Transplantation 78 (2004) 1225–1228.
[9] K. Nakamura, et al., Liver allograft rejection in sensitized recipients. Observations in a clinically relevant small animal model, Am. J. Pathol. 142 (1993) 1383–1391.
[10] A. Yoshizawa, et al., New protocol of immunosuppression for liver transplantation across ABO barrier: the use of rituximab, hepatic arterial infusion, and preservation of spleen, Transplant. Proc. 37 (2005) 1718–1719.
[11] International Panel, Banff schema for grading liver allograft rejection: an international consensus document, Hepatology 25 (1997) 658–663.
[12] D.W. Hanto, et al., ABO-incompatible liver transplantation with no immunological graft losses using total plasma exchange, splenectomy, and quadruple immunosuppression: evidence for accommodation, Liver Transplant. 9 (2003) 22–30.

Kidney transplantation

ELSEVIER

International Congress Series 1292 (2006) 35–41

www.ics-elsevier.com

ABO-incompatible kidney transplantation in Japan

Kazuhide Saito*, Kota Takahashi

Division of Urology, Department of Regenerative and Transplant Medicine, Graduate School of Medical and Dental Sciences, Niigata University, Niigata, Japan
The Japanese ABO-incompatible Kidney Transplantation Committee, Japan

Abstract. Up to 2005, the number of patients on dialysis therapy exceeded more than 250,000 in Japan; however, only 200 deceased and 800 living kidney transplants have been performed annually. We have been making continuous efforts in ABO-incompatible kidney transplantation since 1989 to expand the opportunities for living kidney transplantation in Japan. From the Japanese registry, we have reviewed the long-term patient and graft outcome of ABO-incompatible kidney transplantation. This survey focused on 685 patients who received ABO-incompatible kidney grafts from January 1989 to December 2004 in whom monitoring follow-up could be achieved in 75 institutions. The overall patient survival rates at 1, 3, 5 and 10 years after transplantation were 94%, 91%, 87% and 82%, with overall graft survival rates of 87%, 83%, 76% and 57%, respectively. The graft survival rate was significantly higher in patients aged 29 and younger compared with those aged 30 and older. Especially in children aged 15 and younger, they have shown excellent graft survival rate. The patients with anticoagulation therapy showed significantly higher graft survival rate than those without anticoagulation. There were no significant differences between A- and B-incompatibility with respect to clinical outcomes. There were also no significant difference in numbers of HLA mismatches, induction and maintenance calcinurine inhibitors (ciclosporine vs. tacrolimus) and donor/recipient relationships with respect to the outcomes. A result of most recent 245 cases since 2001 had dramatically improved with 1-year graft survival is 96% and there is a significant difference between the groups in 2001 onwards and before. This study confirms that the outcome of ABO-incompatible living kidney transplantation in Japan is excellent and is similar to that in ABO-compatible cases. ABO-incompatible kidney transplantation has already become one of a standard, safety and effective treatment choice for end-stage renal disease. © 2006 Published by Elsevier B.V.

Keywords: ABO incompatibility; Kidney transplantation; Accommodation

* Corresponding author. Division of Urology, Department of Regenerative and Transplant Medicine, Graduate School of Medical and Dental Sciences, Niigata University, Asahimachi 1-757, Niigata, 951-8510, Japan. Tel.: +81 25 227 2289; fax: +81 25 227 0784.

E-mail address: kazsaito@med.niigata-u.ac.jp (K. Saito).

0531-5131/ © 2006 Published by Elsevier B.V.
doi:10.1016/j.ics.2006.05.004

1. Introduction

Up to 2005, the number of patients on dialysis therapy exceeded 250,000 in Japan and it increases annually by 13,000. However, patients on the waiting list for deceased donor kidney transplantation are only about 12,000. Many patients give up the idea of receiving kidney transplantation because of the very small number of donations. Nowadays in Japan, only about 1000 kidney transplants per year have been performed. Among them, deceased donor kidney transplants are only about 200 per year and 80% are living-related.

For these reasons, we have been making continuous efforts in ABO-incompatible kidney transplantation since 1989 to expand the opportunities for living kidney transplantation in Japan [1–6]. The Japanese ABO-incompatible kidney transplantation committee had started the registry since 1997 [5,6]. In this article, we report the excellent outcome of ABO-incompatible kidney transplantation in Japan on the basis of the recent registry data analysis.

2. Patients and methods

2.1. Patients

Since 1989, 685 of ABO-incompatible kidney transplantations have been performed in 75 institutions up to December 2004; 64% of the recipients were male and 36% female. Their ages ranged from 4 to 71 years, with a mean age of 36.0 years. Most patients were under 50 years of age, but there were about 145 patients (21%) older than 50 years. The mean observation period was 3 years and 4 months (Table 1).

As for the relationship between donors and recipients, parents and children (67%), spouses (15%) were dominant. The number of HLA mismatch was 2.7±1.3.

The blood type O recipients were 55%, type A were 24% and type B were 21%.

2.2. The status of preoperative and postoperative antibody removal

A-incompatible was 51%, B-incompatible was 48% and AB-incompatible was 1%.

Preoperative plasmapheresis was done in 74% and postoperative one was done in 20%.

Table 1

Number of institutions	75
Number of patients	685
Gender	438 (64%) males and 247 (36%) females
Age at operation	mean: 36.0 years old (4–71)
Study period	From January 1989 to December 2004
Period of observation	mean: 3 years 4 months (min. 2 days–max. 15 years and 1 month)
Relationship between donors and recipients	Parents and children: 459 (67%) Spouses: 103 (15%) Siblings: 69 (10%) Others: 54 (8%)
Recipient blood type	A: 166 (24%) B: 144 (21%) O: 375 (55%)
No. of HLA mismatches	2.7±1.3
Plasmapheresis	Pre-operative 505 (74%) Post-operative 134 (20%)
Splenectomy	Yes 610 (89%), No 72 (11%)
Anti-coagulation therapy	Yes 328 (53%), No 287 (47%)
Calcinurine inhibitor	
	Induction CYA 367 (54%), TAC308 (46%), Total $n=564$ Maintenance CYA 336 (51%), TAC317 (49%), Total $n=528$

Preoperative antibody titers were reduced less than 16 times in 56% of recipients in IgM and 45% in IgG, on the other hand, in 14% in IgM and 28% in IgG had exceeded more than 128 times just before transplantation.

2.3. The status of splenectomy and anticoagulation therapy

Up to the end of 2004, splenectomy was performed in 89% of the recipients. 72 (11%) patients who did not undergo splenectomies included those on whom the operation was considered unfeasible, and B-incompatible patients with low antibody titer, or in whom rituximab was used for pre-conditioning regimen. Anti-coagulation therapy was done in about 53% of the patients.

2.4. Immunosuppression therapy

The immunosuppressive therapy commonly used was the triple therapy consisting of a calcinurine inhibitor (CNI) as base, a steroid and an antimetabolite.

For induction, 54% of the patients received ciclosporin and 46% tacrolimus.

For maintenance, 51% received ciclosporin and 49% tacrolimus.

2.5. Control subjects

The control subjects comprised of 1055 patients who received kidney transplantation from living donors at 69 centers in Japan between 1985 and 1995, which included nearly all of centers participated in this study. The clinical characteristics of the control group were similar to those in the patients who received ABO-incompatible kidney transplants as described previously [6].

2.6. Statistical analysis

We analyzed the long-term patient and graft survival by the Kaplan–Meier method and the statistical significance was tested with the use of log-rank tests.

3. Results

3.1. Rejection episodes

Biopsy-proven acute rejection within 3 months after transplantation occurred in 303 cases (47%) of all recipients. After 3 months, biopsy-proven chronic allograft nephropathy had been revealed in 87 (17%) patients among 519 cases who received graft biopsy.

3.2. Patient and graft survival

The overall patient survival rates were of 94%, 91%, 87% and 82% after 1, 3, 5 and 10 years, respectively. The corresponding graft survival rates were of 87%, 83%, 76% and 57%, respectively.

In the historical control of 1055 cases, patient survival rates were of 98%, 97%, 94% and 87%, and graft survival rates were 96%, 89%, 81% and 56%, after 1, 3, 5 and 10 years, respectively.

In the short-term results, the control group showed better results than the ABO-incompatible group. But, in the long-term at 7 and 10 years after transplantation, there was no statistically significant difference between two groups (Fig. 1).

3.3. The graft survival rate by recipient's age

Very good results are shown particularly for pediatric group aged 15 years and younger. Subgroup analysis showed that graft survival rates were significantly higher in 245 recipients aged 29 years and younger (91%, 88%, 81% and 66% at 1, 3, 5 and 10 years, respectively) than in those 440 recipients 30 years and older (85%, 80%, 73% and 50% at 1, 3, 5 and 10 years, respectively) ($p<0.001$, log-rank, Fig. 2).

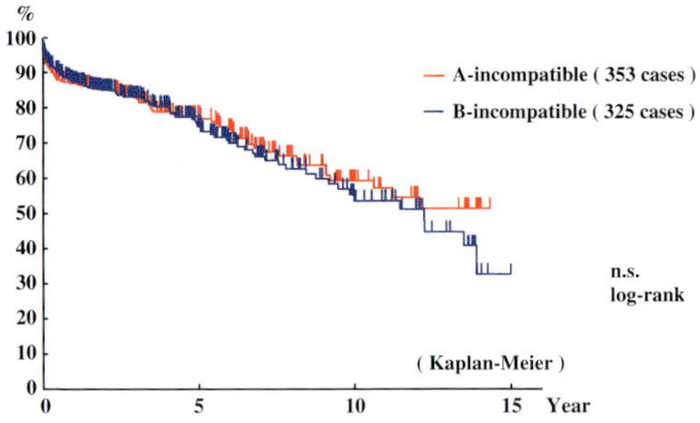

Fig. 5. There was no significant difference in both short-term and long-term graft survival rates between A-incompatible and B-incompatible transplantation.

of living kidney transplantation because of the extreme shortage of the deceased kidney transplants [1–6]. We had settled the Japanese ABO-incompatible kidney transplantation committee and started the registry since 1997 [5,6]. The number of ABO-incompatible transplants gradually increased by year, it has exceeded more than 70 per year recently, which accounts for more than 10% of all the living kidney transplantation in Japan, and overall 685 transplants have been performed in more than 75 institutions up to the end of 2004.

The data had revealed the excellent long-term patient and graft survival as same as those previously reported [5,6], especially 10-year patient and graft survival were as good as those of the historical control living-kidney transplantation. Recipient age and anticoagulation treatment significantly affected the long-term outcome. However, the number of HLA mismatches, A- or B-incompatibility, donor–recipient relationships and induction/maintenance CNI were not the significant factor.

We would like to emphasize the graft survival of 245 cases since 2001 had dramatically improved with one and three-year graft survival is 96% and 94%, respectively. This improvement might be partly due to the use of mycophenolate mofetil (MMF) and anti-CD25 mAb, basiliximab, which had been covered by the Japanese health insurance.

Lessons from our registry data, the onset of antibody mediated rejection (AMR), which has been the major cause of graft loss in the early period after transplant, showed a consistent trend; it occurred within 1 month after transplantation, with a particularly high frequency within the first week, which we think it as a “critical period” of AMR. If the patients had passed uneventfully through the critical period, graft accommodation would be achieved. Antibody removal and regulation of B cell response immediately after transplantation is considered to play a pivotal role in the achievement of accommodation [7–9]. Some centers have adopted a new concept of desensitization therapy started a week or 4 weeks before transplant [10]. Recently, the concept of accommodation and desensitization would make us reconsider the immunosuppression and splenectomy. For more than a decade, splenectomy has been considered to be a necessary prerequisite for successful ABO-incompatible transplantation [6,11]. However, it is already reported that ABO-incompatible kidney transplantation would be carried out successfully without splenectomy using anti-CD20, rituximab, antibody removal and IVIG [12,13]. We have also utilized the desensitization protocol in 13 patients with anti-CD20/MMF/low-dose steroid started 4 weeks before transplantation in ABO-incompatible kidney transplantation without splenectomy since 2004. In this series, we do not perform any additional postoperative antibody removal nor IVIG [14]. High-risk patients, so-called as “high responders” with rebound elevated preoperative antibody titers, may still require splenectomy [15]: however, in most patients, ABO-incompatible kidney transplantation would be safely and successfully performed without splenectomy.

We believe we can completely overcome the ABO-barrier in kidney transplantation in the near future. It would be a great benefit to all the patients waiting for the suitable kidney grafts.

In summary, we conclude that the outcome of ABO-incompatible living kidney transplantation in Japan is excellent and is similar to that in ABO-compatible cases. ABO-incompatible kidney transplantation has already become one of a standard, safety and effective treatment choice for end-stage renal disease.

Acknowledgements

The authors express a special thank to all the members of the Japanese ABO-incompatible transplantation committee, who contributed to this registry. This work was supported in part by a Grant-in-Aid for Research on Human Genome, Tissue Engineering, Food Technology, Health Sciences Research Grants, Ministry of Health, Labor and Welfare of Japan, and by a Grant-in-Aid for Science Research, Ministry of Education and Science of Japan.

References

[1] K. Takahashi, et al., Extracorporeal plasma treatment for extending indication of kidney transplantation: ABO-incompatible and performed antibody-positive kidney transplantation, in: Therapeutic Plasmapheresis, vol. IX, ESAO Press, Cleveland, 1990, pp. 61–63.

[2] K. Takahashi, et al., ABO-incompatible kidney transplantation in a single-center trial, Transplant. Proc. 25 (1993) 271–273.

[3] K. Tanabe, et al., Long-term results of ABO-incompatible living kidney transplantation. A single-center experience, Transplantation 65 (1998) 224–228.

[4] K. Ota, et al., Multicenter trial of ABO-incompatible kidney transplantation, Transpl. Int. 5 (1992) 40–43.

[5] K. Takahashi, et al., First report of a 7-year survey on ABO-incompatible kidney transplantation in Japan, Clin. Exp. Nephrol. 5 (2001) 119–125.

[6] K. Takahashi, et al., Excellent long-term outcome of ABO-incompatible living kidney transplantation in Japan, Am. J. Transp. 4 (2004) 1089–1096.

[7] K. Takahashi, Accommodation in ABO-incompatible kidney transplantation: why do kidney grafts survive? Transplant. Proc. 36 (2004) 193S–196S.

[8] K. Takahashi, Accommodation in ABO-incompatible kidney transplantation—why do kidney grafts survive? Accommodation in ABO-Incompatible Kidney Transplantation, B.V. Elsevier, Amsterdam, 2004, pp. 37–52 Chapter 6.

[9] K. Takahashi, A new concept of accommodation in ABO-incompatible kidney transplantation, Clin. Transplant. 19 (supple. 14) (2005) 76–85.

[10] M. Mannami, N. Mitsuhata, Improved outcomes after ABO-incompatible living-donor kidney transplantation after 4 weeks of treatment with mycophenolate mofetil, Transplantation 79 (2005) 1756–1758.

[11] G.P.J. Alexandre, et al., Splenectomy as a prerequisite for successful human ABO-incompatible renal transplantation, Transplant. Proc. 17 (1985) 138–143.

[12] G. Tyden, G. Kumlien, I. Fehrman, Successful ABO-incompatible kidney transplantations without splenectomy using antigen-specific immunoadsorption and rituximab, Transplantation 76 (2003) 730–743.

[13] C.J. Sonnenday, et al., Plasmapheresis, CMV hyperimmune globulin, and anti-CD20 allow ABO-incompatible renal transplantation without splenectomy, Am. J. Transp. 4 (2004) 1315–1322.

[14] K. Saito, et al., Pinpoint targeted immunosuppression: anti-CD20 /MMF desensitization with anti-CD25 unsuccessful ABO-incompatible kidney transplantation without splenectomy, Xenotransplantation 13 (2006) 111–117.

[15] T. Sawada, S. Fuchinoue, S. Teraoka, Successful A1- to O ABO-incompatible kidney transplantation after a preconditioning regimen consisting of anti-CD20 monoclonal antibody infusions, splenectomy, and double-filtration plasmapheresis, Transplantation 74 (2002) 1207–1210.

ELSEVIER

International Congress Series 1292 (2006) 42–49

www.ics-elsevier.com

Excellent long-term outcomes of ABO-incompatible kidney transplantation in children

Seiichirou Shishido *, Hiroshi Asanuma, Hiroyuki Satoh, Manabu Saneshige, Yoshihito Nanpo

Department of Urology and Kidney Transplantation, Tokyo Metropolitan Kiyose Children's Hospital, Japan

Abstract. Due to profound shortage of suitable deceased allografts, much effort has been made to investigate whether successful kidney transplantation is possible across the ABO blood group barrier even for pediatric recipients. *Methods:* Twenty-five pediatric patients underwent ABO-incompatible living kidney transplantation. All patients received three sessions of plasmapheresis (PP) or immunoadsorption (IA) to remove the anti-A/B antibodies before transplantation. This was followed by splenectomy and a conventional quadruple drug immunosuppressive protocol. To prevent overwhelming postsplenectomy infections, penicillin prophylaxis as well as pretransplant pneumococcal vaccine was given to all patients. *Results:* Of 25 patients, 12 grafts had rebound increases in their anti-A/B isoagglutinin titers within 10 days posttransplant. Moreover, 10 of 12 (83%) patients developed acute rejection with the increase of isoagglutinins. One patient lost the graft because of uncontrolled delayed hyperacute rejection, while the other nine acute rejection episodes were reversed with a standard anti-rejection therapy in combination with PP/IA. Four patients had severe bacterial infectious complications after transplantation. The actuarial 1-, 5- and 10-year graft survival rates are 96%, 91% and 91%, respectively. *Conclusions:* With the adequate desensitization protocol, ABO-incompatible kidney transplantation is a valid alternative even for children with end stage renal disease.

Keywords: ABO-incompatibility; Kidney transplantation; Children; Plasmapheresis; Splenectomy

1. Introduction

Kidney transplantation is now considered as an optimal therapy for all children with end stage renal disease, since it is the only long-term therapy that offers children with chronic renal failure the potential of a near-normal life. However, the current shortage of

* Corresponding author. Tel.: +81 424 91 0011; fax: +81 424 91 0044.
E-mail address: shishido@chp-kiyose-tokyo.jp (S. Shishido).

doi:10.1016/j.ics.2006.03.055

deceased allografts available for transplantation is a global problem. Despite the use of numerous strategies aimed at increasing deceased organ donation, the disparity between organ demand and supply continues to widen.

In addition, patients with blood group B or O are at a disadvantage. According to the United Network of Organ Sharing (UNOS) Scientific Registry, the numbers of patients with blood group A, B, AB and O waiting for kidney transplantation are 18,598 (27.7%), 11,255 (16.8%), 1839 (2.7%) and 35,394 (52.8%), respectively [1].

More importantly, the median waiting times for patients with blood group type B and O are about twice as long as those with blood group type A (740, 1815, 396 and 1469 days for patients with blood group A, B, AB and O, respectively [2]. The percent of kidney registrants transplanted within 1 year of listing ranged by blood type from 9.4% for patients with blood type B to 30.7% for patients with blood type AB; the difference in the percent transplanted for these 2 cohorts is statistically significant [3].

In Japan, where deceased organ donation is limited, more than 80% of pediatric patients receive a kidney from their living relatives. If an appropriate living donor is not available, a child may have to wait for a considerable period of time for a deceased donor. In this setting, blood group ABO incompatibility was regarded as a major obstacle in screening potential living donors [4].

ABO blood type incompatibility between a donor and recipient was generally considered a contraindication to kidney transplantation because of the associated high risk for hyperacute rejection. However, since 1987 when Alexander et al. [5] published a historic series of 23 recipients of ABO-incompatible kidney transplants from living donors, much effort has been made over the last decade to investigate whether successful and effective kidney transplantation is possible across the ABO blood group barrier even in children. In this study, we reviewed our experience with 25 consecutive ABO-incompatible living kidney transplantations in a pediatric population.

2. Materials and methods

2.1. Patients and clinical characteristics

Between 1990 and 2004, 25 pediatric patients underwent ABO-incompatible living kidney transplantation at Tokyo Metropolitan Kiyose Children's Hospital; 20 males and 5 females with a mean ($\pm$ S.D.) age at transplant of 10.6 ± 4.1 years (range 5.9–17.8 years). In each case, the only available living donor was ABO blood group-incompatible. Sixteen patients received living-donor kidney from A1-incompatible donors, while nine patients received kidneys from B-incompatible donors. Donor to recipient ABO blood group antigen incompatibility was as follows: A1 to O in 8; A1B to B in 5; A1 to B in 3; B to O in 7; and A1B to A1 in 2 patients (Table 1). The anti-A or anti-B titer against donor erythrocytes has been determined using the saline method for IgM and the indirect Coombs' test for IgG. Twenty-four patients received a primary kidney graft and one patient had a second transplant.

2.2. Treatment protocol

To remove pre-existing anti-A and/or anti-B antibodies from the recipient's serum prior to kidney transplantation, the initial seven consecutive patients who received ABO-

Table 1
Patient demographics

Gender (male/female)	19/4	
Age at transplantation (year)	10.6 ± 4.1 (5.9–17.8)	
Blood type incompatibility	A1 to O, 8	
	A1B to B, 5	
	A1 to B, 3	
	B to O, 7	
	A1B to A1, 2	
Median pretransplant antibody titers	Anti-A1:	IgM, 1 : 128 (1 : 16–1 : 512)
		IgG, 1 : 32 (1 : 2–1 : 256)
	Anti-B:	IgM, 1 : 32 (1 : 4–1 : 128)
		IgG, 1 : 8 (1 : 2–1 : 128)

incompatible kidney allografts between 1989 and 1993 underwent three sessions of antigen specific immunoadsorption (IA) using Biosynsorb-A or Biosynsorb-B immunoadsorption Column on days 4, 2 and 1 before surgery. Since 1994, a single plasmapheresis (PP) was used with a continuous flow blood cell separator on the same time schedule [4]. In all but the last session, the removed plasma was replaced by 3–5% albumin-containing solution and gamma globulin. During the last PP performed before transplantation, AB blood type fresh-frozen plasma was used as replacement fluid in order to supply complement and clotting factors. Such plasma is also useful to neutralize the remaining isoagglutinin in vivo to reduce anti-A or anti-B IgG and IgM antibody titers. Anti-A/B antibody titers should be reduced to less than 1 : 8 before surgery. Splenectomy was performed at the time of transplantation.

Our current posttransplant immunosuppressive protocol for pediatric kidney transplantation across the ABO barrier was a quadruple drug regimen with cyclosporine (CsA), methylprednisolone, cyclophosphamide and antilymphocyte globulin (ALG) or deoxyspergualine (DSG). Cyclophosphamide was given to suppress the production of anti-A/B antibodies for 10 days prior to transplantation, and was switched to mycophenolate mofetil (MMF) at 2 months posttransplant.

CsA was given for 3 days at 70 mg/m^2 i.v. every 12 h postoperatively, followed by oral CsA (350 mg/m^2), aiming at AUC0–4 of 4000–5000 ng/h/ml for the first month, 3500 ng/h/ml for the second month, and 2500 ng/h/ml thereafter. The initial dose of methylprednisolone was 40 mg/m^2/day with taper.

Dipyridamole (5 mg/kg) and ticlopidine hydrochloride (5 mg/kg) were administered, starting 4 days posttransplantation to prevent platelet aggregation. To prevent the overwhelming postsplenectomy infection, penicillin prophylaxis as well as pneumococcal vaccination is given to all recipients of any age group at least for 12 months. Furthermore, younger recipients receive the penicillin prophylaxis up to 10 years of age.

2.3. Statistical methods

Allograft and patient survival rates were calculated using the Kaplan–Meyer method. Statistical analysis was performed using the commercially available software, StatView J-7.0 (SAS Institute Inc. USA).

3. Results

The patients were followed from 6 to 189 months with a mean follow-up of 90 months.

Median pretransplant anti-A1 antibody titers in 16 recipients incompatible for blood group A antigens were 1 : 128 in IgM (range 1 : 16–1 : 512) and 1 : 32 in IgG (range 1 : 2–1 : 256), while the median anti-B titers in 9 blood group B-incompatible recipients were 1 : 32 in IgM (range 1 : 4–1 : 128) and 1 : 8 in IgG (range 1 : 2–1 : 128). Fourteen of 25 (56%) patients had a high (≥ 1 : 64) pretransplant anti-A or anti-B isoagglutinin titer.

All recipients who underwent ABO-incompatible renal transplantation achieved a pretransplant isoagglutinin titer less than 1 : 8 with 3 to 4 sessions of PP/IA treatment. No patients developed adverse effects related to PP/IA therapy.

Splenectomy was performed on all recipients at the time of transplantation. There were no surgical complications of splenectomy. All patients had evidence of immediate graft function.

Of the 25 patients, 12 grafts (9 of 16 cases with blood group A-incompatible grafts and 3 of 9 cases with blood group B antigen-incompatible grafts) had rebound increases in their IgM and/or IgG anti-A and/or anti-B titers to greater than 1 : 64 or predepletion levels within 10 days posttransplant (median 7 days). Furthermore, 10 of 12 (83%) patients developed acute rejection with such rebound increases of isoagglutinin titers. One patient who received an A1 antigen-positive kidney lost the graft with a marked rebound increase in IgM and IgG anti-A1 titers 5 days posttransplant. Pathological examination was consistent with hyperacute rejection. Whilst the other nine patients who developed acute rejection in association with the increase in their antibody titers were successfully treated by a combination of high dose steroid therapy and one to three sessions of PP or IA (mean: 1.6 sessions per patient). After the third week posttransplant, only 3 patients had acute rejection. There was no correlation between the development of rejection and their isoagglutinin titers. These were reversed with a course of pulse steroid therapy. The total rate of acute rejection was 48%, which is not different from that of ABO-compatible kidney transplantation.

Four patients had severe bacterial infectious complications after transplantation. Three patients developed *Klebsiella pneumoniae* sepsis within 3 months posttransplant, which was treated successfully with antibiotics. One patient had an episode of bacterial otitis media, and was treated with open drainage of his eardrum and antibiotics. Lower urinary tract infections were also seen in 3 other patients.

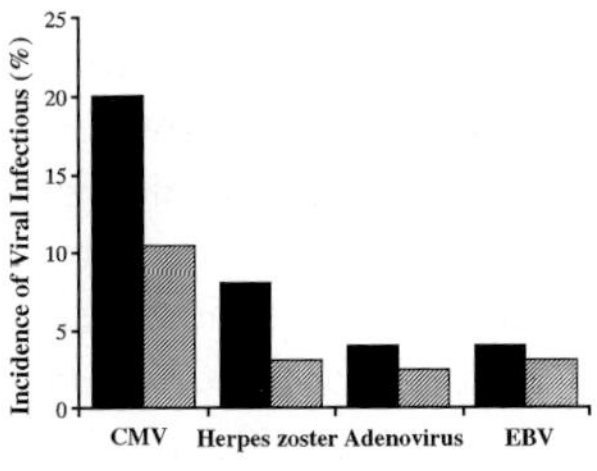

Fig. 1. The incidence of virus infection in patients with ABO-incompatible kidney transplantation (black bars) and ABO-incompatible kidney transplantation (striped bars).

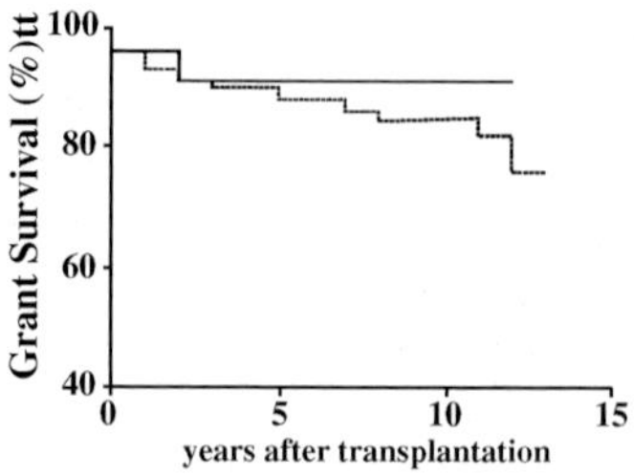

Fig. 2. Graft survival in recipients with ABO-incompatible (solid line) and ABO-compatible (dotted line) grafts.

Cytomegalovirus (CMV) infection was the most frequent infection and occurred in 5 (20%) patients. However, no patient had a serious tissue-invasive CMV disease. Herpes zoster infection occurred in two patients and successfully treated with acyclovir. EB virus infection and adenovirus infection was also noted in one patient each. Fortunately, no patient developed EBV-related PTLD. The incidence of virus infection in the ABO-incompatible kidney transplantation was not different compared with those of ABO-compatible transplantation (Fig. 1).

Patient survival is 100% to date. The actuarial 1-, 5- and 10-year graft survival rates are 96%, 91% and 91%, respectively. As shown in Fig. 2, there is no significant difference in the long-term graft outcome between ABO-compatible and -incompatible transplantation.

4. Discussion

This report describes our 15 years' experience of ABO-incompatible living-donor kidney transplantation in children. The basic pre- and posttransplant sensitization protocol in a pediatric recipient is almost the same as those in an adult patient. The protocol consists of preoperative PP, four-drug immunosuppression and concomitant splenectomy. Our data clearly demonstrate that this protocol can lead to successful long-term results even in a pediatric population.

In order to prevent hyperacute rejection due to pre-existing anti-A and/or anti-B antibodies reacting with vascular endothelium, it is necessary to remove these antibodies from the recipient's serum prior to kidney transplantation.

A single PP with a filtration technique is the most commonly used technique for antibody reduction in children. In our current protocol, we mostly use a single PP with a continuous flow blood cell separator on days 4, 2, and 1 before surgery. Double filtration plasmapheresis (DFPP), which was developed to minimize the volume of substitution fluid, is the most popular plasma filtration method for the treatment of adults [6]. This procedure is also effective for pediatric patients. However, care should be taken with small children to ensure that they do not develop hypervolemia and hypoalbuminemia. Antigen-specific immunoadsorption (IA) is also effective at removing anti-A and/or anti-B antibodies even in younger recipients. In our series, the initial seven consecutive patients who received ABO-incompatible kidney allografts between 1989 and 1993 underwent three sessions of antigen specific IA using Biosynsorb-A or Biosynsorb-B-immunoadsorption Column on the same time schedule. However, this procedure is not used at present in our country since the use of Biosynsorb Column mentioned above was not approved by the National Health Insurance of Japan due to its significant expense. Therefore, in our present protocol, we use single PP as previously outlined [4].

The basic immunosuppressive protocol in a pediatric recipient is almost the same as in an adult patient. Regarding the posttransplant immunosuppression, it has been generally thought that the initial immunosuppression for ABO-incompatible kidney transplant recipients should be more rigorous than those for ABO-compatible transplants in order to avoid antibody-mediated rejection [7]. Tanabe and Ohta et al. [6,8] used a quintuple drug regimen consisting of CsA/tacrolimus, azathioprine, steroids, ALG and DSG with splenectomy and local irradiation of the donor graft for their ABO-incompatible kidney transplant recipients including pediatric cases. Our current protocol for pediatric kidney transplantation across the ABO barrier was a quadruple drug regimen with CsA, methylprednisolone, cyclophosphamide and DSG. Cyclophosphamide was given to suppress the production of anti-A/B antibodies for 10 days prior to transplantation and was switched to MMF at 2 months posttransplant.

There is still some controversy regarding the necessity of splenectomy in ABO-incompatible living kidney transplantation. Several previous studies demonstrated that the spleen played a major role in the production of anti-A/anti-B antibodies and was likely to be involved in the initiation of the early stages of humoral rejection. Therefore, splenectomy has been considered an essential procedure for successful ABO-incompatible kidney transplantation at many transplant centers [5,6].

Indeed surgical splenectomy provides efficacious treatment for preventing antibody mediated rejection, but it is also associated with perioperative morbidity and a life-long risk of overwhelming infections. The risk is highest in infant and young children, but adults also have an increased risk of infection [9]. In a review of over 12,000 patients who had undergone splenectomy, the incidence of serious post-splenectomy infections was found to be 15.7% in infants, 10.7% in children under the age of 5 years, and 0.9% in adults [10]. Furthermore, the risk of splenectomy may be even greater in immunosuppressed patients after transplantation [11].

These infections are most often due to encapsulated organisms, especially pneumococcus, *Haemophilus influenzae* type B, and meningococcus, but any bacterial agent may cause the rapid onset of septicemia, meningitis, pneumonia and shock characteristic of the asplenic condition [7]. Preventing strategies are very important and fall into three major categories: immunoprophylaxis, antibiotic prophylaxis and education. The efficacy of pneumococcal vaccination in preventing infection has been demonstrated in children with splenectomy. In addition, the use of long-term penicillin prophylaxis is also recommended in asplenic children in order to prevent pneumococcal infection [12]. In our current protocol, penicillin prophylaxis as well as pneumococcal vaccination is given to all ABO-incompatible kidney transplant recipients of any age group at least for 12 months. Furthermore, younger recipients receive the penicillin prophylaxis up to 10 years of age.

Several recent studies have demonstrated that ABO-incompatible kidney transplantation can be performed without splenectomy with excellent results, using an infusion of rituximab, a chimeric murine/human monoclonal antibody directed against the CD20 antigen, in combination with PP/IA [13,14]. Sonnenday et al. [14] suggested that because of the benefit of splenectomy appears to be greatest in the early month posttransplant, a transient biological splenectomy created with the use of rituximab would allow protection against excess early graft loss due to antibody-mediated rejection, while avoiding the long-term risks of splenectomy. Since young recipients undergoing splenectomy are at a greater risk of serious infections, we should further study a new splenectomy avoidance protocol for pediatric patients who receive ABO-incompatible kidney allografts.

Except for the bacterial infections mentioned above, viral infection, most commonly CMV and opportunistic infection with *Pneumocystis carinii*, *Listeria monocytogenes* and *Aspergillus fumigatus*, are common after the second month posttransplant [7]. CMV infection is an important source of morbidity and mortality in transplant recipients. Patients who experience primary CMV infection at the time of transplantation are at the highest risk of clinically significant CMV disease. Since a higher percentage of young pediatric recipients are CMV-negative at the time of transplantation, transplantation of a kidney from a CMV-positive donor into a CMV negative recipient is associated with a significant incidence of posttransplant primary CMV infection. Appropriate prophylaxis, by anti-CMV IgG or ganciclovir/acyclovir, is warranted in the child at risk for primary infection [15].

In the current study, we showed excellent long-term outcomes in pediatric recipients who received kidney transplantation across the ABO barrier. The long-term patient and graft survival rates were comparable with the rates for patients undergoing ABO-compatible kidney allografts. According to the pooled analysis of ABO-incompatible kidney transplantations in Japan [16], results are extremely favorable in children up to 15 years of age, with a graft survival rate of 90% at 1 year, 85% at 5 years and 76% at 9 years. Results are also good for patients 16 to 29 years of age, with a graft survival rate of 90% at 1 year, 76% at 5 years and 74% at 9 years. These data clearly show that young recipients may be better candidates for ABO-incompatible living-donor kidney transplantations.

The exact mechanisms responsible for the fact that the younger children respond better compared with adults are unknown. Most pediatric patients received a kidney allograft from their young and healthy parents. Therefore, such kidney allografts may respond less to immunologic and non-immunologic stress. Otherwise, these data may suggest that the pediatric immune system is less prone to antibody-mediated rejection.

5. Conclusion

We have demonstrated that with adequate pretransplant depletion of pre-existing anti-A and/or anti-B antibodies by PP/IA and splenectomy, followed by a quadruple drug immunosuppressive regimen being reinforced with ALG/DSG, successful kidney transplantation is possible across the ABO barrier even for children with end stage renal disease. All recipients achieved a pretransplant isoagglutinin titer less than 1 : 8 with 3 to 4 sessions of PP/IA treatment. No patient developed adverse effects related to PP/IA therapy. In addition, there were no surgical complications of splenectomy. We also showed that posttransplant PP combined with anti-rejection therapy was effective for patients who had an early acute rejection in association with rebound increases in anti-A and/or anti-B titers. No significant difference in the incidence of infectious complication between ABO-incompatible and ABO-compatible kidney transplantation. The use of a pretransplant pneumococcal vaccine and long-term penicillin prophylaxis could be effective in preventing overwhelming postsplenectomy infection. The long-term patient and graft outcome of ABO-incompatible living kidney transplantation is excellent and comparable with that of ABO-compatible transplantations.

References

[1] UNOS, Annual Report of the US Scientific Registry of Transplant Recipients and the Organ Procurement and Transplantation Network, United Network for Organ Sharing, Richmond, VA, 2005.

[2] The U.S. Organ Procurement and Transplantation Network and the Scientific Registry of Transplant Recipients OPTN/SRTR Annual Report.

[3] M.A. McBride, A.M. Harper, S.E. Taranto, The OPTN Waiting List, 1988–2002, in: Checa, Terasaki (Eds.), Clin. Transplant. 2003, UCLA Immunogenetics Center, Los Angeles, 2003, pp. 53–64.

[4] S. Shishido, et al., ABO-incompatible living-donor kidney transplantation in children, Transplantation 72 (2001) 1037–1042.

[5] G.P.J. Alexandre, et al., Present experiences in a series of 26 ABO-incompatible living donor renal allografts, Transplant. Proc. 19 (1987) 4538–4542.

[6] K. Tanabe, et al., Long-term results of ABO-incompatible living kidney transplantation, Transplantation 65 (1998) 224–228.

[7] S. Shishido, A. Hasegawa, Current status of ABO-incompatible kidney transplantation in children, Pediatr. Transplant. 9 (2005) 148–154.

[8] T. Ohta, et al., ABO-incompatible pediatric kidney transplantation in a single-center trial, Pediatr. Nephrol. 14 (2000) 1–5.

[9] D.C. Melles, S. de Marie, Prevention of infection in hyposplenic and asplenic patients: an update, Neth. J. Med. 62 (2004) 45–52.

[10] R. Holdsworth, A. Irving, A. Cuschieri, Postsplenectomy sepsis and its mortality rate: acute versus perceived risks, Br. J. Surg. 78 (1991) 1031–1038.

[11] J.W. Alexander, et al., The late adverse effect of splenectomy on patient survival following cadaveric renal transplantation, Transplantation 37 (1984) 467–470.

[12] E. Castagnola, F. Fioredda, Prevention of life-threatening infections due to encapsulated bacteria in children with hyposplenia or asplenia: a brief review of current recommendations for practical purpose, Eur. J. Haematol. 71 (2003) 319–326.

[13] G. Tyden, et al., ABO incompatible kidney transplantation without splenectomy, using antigen-specific immunoadsorption and rituximab, Am. J. Transp. 5 (1) (2005) 145–148.

[14] C.J. Sonnenday, et al., Plasmapheresis, CMV hyperimmune globulin, and anti-CD20 allow ABO-incompatible renal transplantation without splenectomy, Am. J. Transp. 4 (8) (2004) 1315–1322.

[15] G. Bock, E.K. Sullivan, D. Miller, Cytomegalovirus infections following renal transplantation – effects on antiviral prophylaxis: a Report of the North American Pediatric Renal Transplant Cooperative Study, Pediatr. Nephrol. 11 (1997) 665–671.

[16] K. Takahashi, et al., Excellent long-term outcome of ABO-incompatible living donor kidney transplantation in Japan, Am. J. Transp. 4 (2004) 1089–1096.

Liver transplantation

ELSEVIER

International Congress Series 1292 (2006) 53–60

www.ics-elsevier.com

ABO-incompatible transplantation: Accommodation by upregulation of protective genes — A hypothesis

Douglas W. Hanto *

Beth Israel Deaconess Medical Center, Harvard Medical School, USA

Abstract. ABO-incompatible kidney and liver transplants can be performed successfully by depleting anti-A or anti-B isoagglutinins pretransplant and by suppressing their development posttransplant. With these protocols, humoral rejection can be avoided. Recovery of isohemagglutinin antibody levels without humoral rejection suggests accommodation, the ability of an organ allograft to survive in the presence of anti-graft antibodies and complement, may be the protective mechanism preventing late antibody-mediated rejection. This may be related to the ability of endothelial cells, the target of antibody-mediated rejection, to upregulate protective genes, including those encoding heme oxygenase-1 (HO-1) that then block the proinflammatory response of the endothelial cells and thereby rejection. Induced expression of HO-1 in the endothelial cells of the graft before transplantation may prevent apoptosis of those cells after transplantation, and prevent the generation of endothelial cell-based inflammation that leads to rejection. Experimental and clinical studies in ABO-incompatible models will be required to examine this hypothesis, and determine whether carbon monoxide (CO) might be able to modulate antibody-mediated rejection after ABO-incompatible transplantation. © 2006 Published by Elsevier B.V.

Keywords: ABO-incompatible transplantation; Accommodation; Heme oxygenase-1; Protective genes

1. Introduction

ABO-incompatible kidney and liver transplants are now performed with success rates approaching those of ABO-compatible transplants. Because antibody-mediated rejection of ABO-incompatible transplants can be caused by anti-A or anti-B isohemagglutinins, protocols have been developed to deplete these antibodies pretransplant and to suppress their development posttransplant. In ABO-incompatible kidney transplants, the risk of

* 110 Francis Street, 7th Floor, Boston, USA.
E-mail address: dhanto@bidmc.harvard.edu.

0531-5131/ © 2006 Published by Elsevier B.V.
doi:10.1016/j.ics.2006.03.060

antibody-mediated rejection can be reduced by pre- and post-transplant total plasma exchange (TPE), splenectomy, and induction immunosuppression that often includes a polyclonal or monoclonal anti-T cell antibody [1–4]. Protocols have also been developed which include pre- and post-transplant TPE, but substitute anti-CD20 monoclonal antibody and IVIG (intravenous immune globulin) for splenectomy, and in some cases avoid antibody induction [5–9].

In ABO-incompatible liver transplants, antibody-mediated rejection has been associated with a high risk of vascular thrombosis and ischemic bile duct complications that led to poor patient and graft survival rates [10]. With pre- and post-transplant TPE, splenectomy and monoclonal antibody induction, antibody-mediated rejection can be eliminated, along with vascular and biliary complications, leading to patient and graft survival rates that are comparable with ABO-compatible transplants [11–13]. ABO-incompatible living donor liver transplants have also been done successfully, primarily in Japan where deceased donor organs are not as available [14,15]. ABO-incompatible heart transplants can be performed successfully in infants before isohemagglutinin production begins, usually at 12 to 14 months [16].

2. ABO-incompatible liver transplantation

2.1. Clinical protocol

We have used a protocol in ABO-incompatible deceased donor liver transplant recipients that includes: pretransplant TPE to remove anti-A and anti-B isohemagglutinins; posttransplant TPE to maintain low titers for 2 weeks posttransplant; splenectomy at the time of transplantation and the administration of cytoxan or mycophenolate mofetil to reduce antibody production; and quadruple immunosuppression to reduce the risk of cellular rejection and to decrease antibody production [11]. The donor/recipient blood type combinations were: A_1 to O in 7, B to O in 2, B to A in 2, A to B in 1, AB to A in 1, and AB to O in 1. All patients except one underwent pretransplant double volume TPE (which removes 90% of the Ig) using plasma that was ABO-compatible with both the patient serum and the donor liver. O recipients received fresh frozen plasma of the donor type (A or B), A recipients of B and AB livers received AB plasma, and B and O recipients of AB livers received AB plasma. The anti-A and anti-B isohemagglutinin titers were assessed pretransplant and daily for the first 2 weeks posttransplant.

2.2. Summary of results

Actuarial 1- and 5-year patient and graft survival rates were 71.4% and 61.2% and 71.4% and 61.2%, respectively, with a mean follow-up of 62.9 ± 39.4 months. Seven patients developed 10 episodes of acute cellular rejection, and the mean time to the first episode was 62 ± 33 days. There were no antibody-mediated rejection episodes or vascular thromboses. Pretransplant and pre-TPE IgG mean isohemagglutinin titers were 262 ± 326 compared with pretransplant post-TPE titers of 65 ± 103 ($p=0.04$) with 8 of 9 patients with measurable titers pre- and post-TPE achieving a reduction in titers (Table 1). The mean number of posttransplant TPE was 5.5 ± 4.1 (range 0–12), and the last TPE was on postoperative day 9.4 ± 5.3. IgG isohemagglutinin titers 2 weeks posttransplant had increased to 153 ± 309 ($p=0.03$ compared with pretransplant pre-TPE IgG).

Table 1
Isoagglutinin titers[a] pre- and post-TPE

Patient	Isoagglutinin titer	1 Pre-TX Pre-TPE IgM	2 Pre-TX Pre-TPE IgG	3 Pre-TX Post-TPE IgM	4 Pre-TX Post-TPE IgG	5 # Pre-Tx TPE	6 # Post-Tx TPE	7 POD # of last TPE	8 Two weeks post-Tx IgM	9 Two weeks post-Tx IgG
1	Anti-B	64	64	4	4	1	5	9	2	32
2[b]	*	*	*	*	*	*	*	*	*	*
3	Anti-A	64	512	32	256	1	6	5	32	128
4	Anti-B	64	32	ND	ND	0	9	15	4	16
5	Anti-A	8	128	8	64	1	0	–	0	2
6	Anti-A	32	256	4	32	1	0	–	8	16
7	Anti-B	16	32	1	8	1	10	16	32	64
8	Anti-B	8	16	4	16	1	9	15	8	32
9[b]	*	*	*	*	*	*	*	*	*	*
10	Anti-B	8	8	ND	ND	1	1	1	1	<1
11[b]	*	*	*	*	*	*	*	*	*	*
12	Anti-A	ND	512	ND	4	1	12	12	ND	4
13	Anti-A	ND	1024	ND	256	1	6	6	ND	1024
	Anti-B	ND	512	ND	4				ND	512
14	Anti-A	ND	16	ND	2	1	3	6	ND	2
Mean ± S.D.		33 ± 27	262 ± 326	8.8 ± 11.6	65 ± 103		5.5 ± 4.1	9.4 ± 5.3	10.9 ± 13.4	153 ± 309

P values: 1 vs. 3 = 0.03; 1 vs. 8 = 0.06; 2 vs. 4 = 0.04; 2 vs. 9 = 0.03; 3 vs. 8 = 0.38; 4 vs. 9 = 0.20.

Reprinted from Hanto et al. [11] with permission.

[a] Titers are expressed as the reciprocal of the titer.

2.3. Discussion

ABO-incompatible deceased donor liver transplantation historically led to antibody-mediated rejection, poor patient and graft survival, and vascular thrombosis and ischemic bile duct complications. Farges et al. [10] reported on 40 patients with 1- and 5-year patient survival rates of 52% and 50% and graft survival rates of 30% and 20%, respectively. Immunohistologic findings were consistent with antibody-mediated rejection and there was a higher risk of arterial thromboses and delayed bile duct strictures and cholangitis in surviving patients. Nine patients received plasmapheresis posttransplant, whereas none were treated pretransplant, and nine received quadruple immunosuppression, but their analysis did not allow conclusions to be drawn regarding the effectiveness of these modalities. Mor et al. [17] reported an improvement in results in 8 adult and 2 pediatric patients using quadruple therapy and pretransplant plasmapheresis in selected patients. Six of eight adults (75%) were alive at the time of the report and 4/8 (50%) grafts were still functioning. However, three adult patients (37.5%) lost their grafts to antibody-mediated rejection at 5, 12, and 30 days posttransplant.

By utilizing all modalities including pre- and post-TPE, splenectomy and quadruple immunosuppressive therapy, we have achieved acceptable patient and graft survival rates. The patient deaths were reflective of the type of seriously ill patient generally considered for an ABO-incompatible transplant, but had nothing to do with the ABO incompatibility itself. Three of the four early deaths were in the higher risk older age category, all being 60 years of age or older. If these perioperative deaths are excluded both the 1- and 5-year patient survival rates and graft survival rates were 100% and 85.7%, respectively. We had no graft losses due to antibody-mediated rejection and no increased incidence of vascular or biliary tract complications. These results represent a significant improvement over those previously reported as noted above.

There may be several reasons for these results. First, all patients underwent pre- and post-transplant double-volume TPE which removes 90% of circulating Ig, whereas a single-volume TPE removes only 67%. In prior reports patients received either no TPE, only posttransplant TPE, or 1–1.5 volume TPE pre- and post-transplant in selected patients, but not all [10,17]. We attempted to keep the isohemagglutinin titer ≤ 1 : 8, or as low as possible during the first 2 weeks posttransplant and TPE was very effective in reducing the pretransplant IgG titers in 89% of patients with 56% achieving the goal of a titer ≤ 1 : 8. It is unclear, however, from published data or our data how frequently TPE should be performed or for how long. It is also unclear what an optimal target titer is. Some guidelines and conclusions can be drawn from our data and have been previously published [11]. Some patients required no or one posttransplant TPE because of either a low initial titer or a high pretransplant titer that responded to TPE and remained low posttransplant. A second group had low IgG titers that responded well to TPE, but required multiple posttransplant TPE to maintain low titers. A third group had high titers that required multiple posttransplant TPE, but the titers could be reduced to desired levels in only one patient. In spite of the high titers in the third group, humoral rejection still did not occur. This may be in part related to the removal of significant quantities of antibody and complement by TPE. In addition, the liver appears to be able to tolerate higher titers, a finding that may be related to its ability to absorb antibodies. The duration and frequency of TPE should be individualized based on titers and response to TPE, but a maximum of 14 days of TPE appears to be adequate.

All patients except one underwent splenectomy whereas splenectomy was not performed in the other series of ABO-incompatible liver transplants [10,17]. Splenectomy has routinely been performed in ABO-incompatible kidney transplantation in order to reduce antibody formation and decrease the risk of hyperacute rejection. However, recent studies in ABO-incompatible kidney transplants have shown that anti-CD20 monoclonal antibody therapy can safely substitute for splenectomy [5–8]. Splenectomy continues to be used in living donor adult liver transplantation [14,18], although it has been combined with anti-CD20 in some cases [13]. Splenectomy has not been used routinely in pediatric ABO-incompatible liver transplants because pediatric patients have lower natural titers of alloantibodies and are at greater risk for overwhelming postsplenectomy sepsis.

Patients received induction immunosuppression in our series with cytoxan or mycophenolate mofetil which can block antibody production, along with steroids, cyclosporine, and OKT3, the latter of which theoretically can block T cell-dependent B-cell antibody production. No patient developed humoral rejection. Mor et al. [17] used cytoxan, prednisone, OKT3, and Neoral, but did not splenectomize any patient but only used TPE selectively and had a 30% early graft loss due to humoral rejection. Thus, the immunosuppressive regimen is an adjunct, but not a substitute for TPE and splenectomy. Novel immunosuppressive therapies such as portal vein infusion with methylprednisolone, prostaglandin E1, and gabexate mesilate have also been utilized successfully [18].

2.4. Conclusion

ABO-incompatible liver transplants can be performed with acceptable patient and graft survival rates with a low risk of antibody-mediated rejection with a combination of TPE, splenectomy and quadruple immunosuppression. Recovery of isohemagglutinin antibody levels without humoral rejection suggests accommodation may be the protective mechanism preventing late antibody-mediated rejection.

3. Accommodation

3.1. Clinical relevance

Clinical studies have focused on maintaining low isohemagglutinin titers for 2 weeks posttransplantation, after which the allograft seems to be resistant to increases in isohemagglutinin antibody titers. This is a clinical example of the immunological phenomenon called accommodation that refers to the ability of an organ allograft to survive in the presence of anti-graft antibodies and complement. This may be related to the ability of endothelial cells, the target of antibody-mediated rejection, to upregulate protective genes, including those encoding hemoxygenase-1, A20, Bcl-2 and Bcl-x_L, that then block the proinflammatory response of the endothelial cells and thereby rejection [19,20]. One of these genes, heme oxygenase-1 (HO-1), has been of particular interest [21].

3.2. Xenotransplantation model

Accommodation has been studied in xenotransplantation models that have relevance to ABO-incompatible transplantation. The transplantation of hamster hearts into rats that have been sensitized to hamster cardiac grafts leads to hyperacute rejection. Complement depletion with cobra venom factor (CVF) and cyclosporine prevents hyperacute rejection, but the grafts undergo delayed antibody-mediated rejection. By removing pre-existing antibody and slowing the rate of return of antibody by blood exchange, CVF, cyclosporine, cytoxan and splenectomy, long-term survival of the grafts can be achieved [19]. These grafts survive in the presence of anti-donor IgM, IgG, and complement. The surviving hearts express high levels of the protective genes A20, Bcl-2, Bcl-x_L and HO-1 in their endothelial cells and smooth muscle cells.

3.3. Heme oxygenase-1 (HO-1)

HO-1 catabolizes heme into carbon monoxide (CO), biliverdin, and free iron (Fe^{2+}). It functions as a protective gene because of its anti-inflammatory and anti-apoptotic properties and its anti-proliferative effects on endothelial, epithelial and smooth muscle cells. In a model of mouse-to-rat cardiac xenografts, rapid HO-1 expression by endothelial cells, smooth muscle cells, and cardiac myocytes is necessary for protection of the xenografts from rejection [20].

3.4. Carbon monoxide (CO)

CO has also been shown to cytoprotective in several rodent disease models including a mouse cardiac xenotransplantation model and can substitute for HO-1 [20,21]. It has been shown that mouse hearts transplanted into normal rats treated with CVF and cyclosporine survive indefinitely. If the hearts are unable to express HO-1, because they lack the gene encoding HO 1 (*hmox*$^{-/-}$) or HO-1 activity is suppressed by tin protoporphyrin, they are rejected. If the heart is unable to express HO-1 and both the donor and recipient are treated with CO, the hearts survive indefinitely (Fig. 1). CO has the ability to block the proinflammatory, and enhances the anti-inflammatory response of monocytes and macrophages. CO also: (1) inhibits platelet activation and aggregation which blocks thrombosis and the pro-inflammatory response induced by activated platelets; (2) inhibits the expression of plasminogen activator inhibitor type 1 (PAI-1) that blocks ischemia

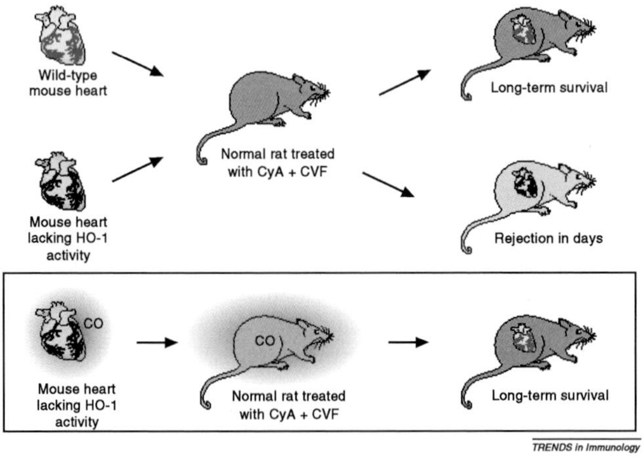

Fig. 1. HO-1 requirement for graft survival can be replaced by CO. From Otterbein et al. [21] with permission.

reperfusion; (3) blocks apoptosis in endothelial cells, fibroblasts, hepatocytes, and β-cells [21]. CO can also suppress chronic rejection [22].

3.5. Hypothesis

It is hypothesized that accommodation is achieved because the protective genes protect the endothelial cells from apoptosis and suppress the pro-inflammatory response of endothelial cells to stimuli such as antibody plus complement. Induced expression of HO-1 in the endothelial cells of the graft before transplantation may prevent apoptosis of those cells after transplantation and prevent the generation of endothelial cell-based inflammation that leads to rejection. Furthermore, clinical and experimental studies in ABO-incompatible models will be required to examine this hypothesis and determine whether CO might be able to modulate antibody-mediated rejection after ABO-incompatible transplantation.

References

[1] J.M. Gloor, et al., ABO-incompatible kidney transplantation using both A2 and non-A2 living donors, Transplantation 75 (7) (2003) 971–977.
[2] M.D. Stegall, P.G. Dean, J.M. Gloor, ABO-incompatible kidney transplantation, Transplantation 78 (5) (2004) 635–640.
[3] K. Takahashi, et al., Excellent long-term outcome of ABO-incompatible living donor kidney transplantation in Japan, Am. J. Transp. 4 (7) (2004) 1089–1096.
[4] K. Tanabe, et al., Long-term results of ABO-incompatible living kidney transplantation: a single-center experience, Transplantation 65 (2) (1998) 224–228.
[5] G. Tyden, et al., ABO incompatible kidney transplantations without splenectomy, using antigen-specific immunoadsorption and rituximab, Am. J. Transp. 5 (1) (2005) 145–148.
[6] G. Tyden, G. Kumlien, I. Fehrman, Successful ABO-incompatible kidney transplantations without splenectomy using antigen-specific immunoadsorption and rituximab, Transplantation 76 (4) (2003) 730–731.
[7] C.J. Sonnenday, et al., Plasmapheresis, CMV hyperimmune globulin, and anti-CD20 allow ABO-incompatible renal transplantation without splenectomy, Am. J. Transpl. 4 (8) (2004) 1315–1322.
[8] D.L. Segev, et al., ABO incompatible high-titer renal transplantation without splenectomy or anti-CD20 treatment, Am. J. Transp. 5 (10) (2005) 2570–2575.
[9] J.M. Gloor, et al., A comparison of splenectomy versus intensive posttransplant antidonor blood group antibody monitoring without splenectomy in ABO-incompatible kidney transplantation, Transplantation 80 (11) (2005) 1572–1577.
[10] O. Farges, et al., The use of ABO-incompatible grafts in liver transplantation: a life-saving procedure in highly selected patients, Transplantation 59 (8) (1995) 1124–1133.
[11] D.W. Hanto, et al., ABO-incompatible liver transplantation with no immunological graft losses using total plasma exchange, splenectomy, and quadruple immunosuppression: evidence for accommodation, Liver Transplant. 9 (1) (2003) 22–30.
[12] M. Stegall, ABO-incompatible liver transplant: is it justifiable? Liver Transplant. 9 (1) (2003) 31.
[13] M. Usuda, et al., Successful use of anti-CD20 monoclonal antibody (rituximab) for ABO-incompatible living-related liver transplantation, Transplantation 79 (1) (2005) 12–16.
[14] H. Sekido, et al., Successful adult ABO-incompatible liver transplantation: therapeutic strategy for thrombotic microangiopathy is the key to success, Transplantation 75 (9) (2003) 1605–1607.
[15] M. Shimazu, M. Kitajima, Living donor liver transplantation with special reference to ABO incompatible grafts and small-for-size grafts, World J. Surg. 28 (1) (2004) 2–7.
[16] L.J. West, et al., ABO-incompatible heart transplantation in infants, N. Engl. J. Med. 344 (11) (2001) 793–800.
[17] E. Mor, et al., Successful use of an enhanced immunosuppressive protocol with plasmapheresis for ABO-incompatible mismatched grafts in liver transplant recipients, Transplantation 59 (7) (1995) 986–990.

[18] M. Tanabe, et al., Intraportal infusion therapy as a novel approach to adult ABO-incompatible liver transplantation, Transplantation 73 (12) (2002) 1959–1961.
[19] Y. Lin, et al., Long-term survival of hamster hearts in presensitized rats, J. Immunol. 164 (9) (2000) 4883–4892.
[20] M.P. Soares, et al., Expression of heme oxygenase-1 can determine cardiac xenograft survival, Nat. Med. 4 (9) (1998) 1073–1077.
[21] L.E. Otterbein, et al., Heme oxygenase-1: unleashing the protective properties of heme, Trends Immunol. 24 (8) (2003) 449–455.
[22] L.E. Otterbein, et al., Carbon monoxide suppresses arteriosclerotic lesions associated with chronic graft rejection and with balloon injury, Nat. Med. 9 (2) (2003) 183–190.

Lung transplantation

International Congress Series 1292 (2006) 63–69

www.ics-elsevier.com

ABO-incompatible lung transplantation

R.N. Pierson [a,*], J. Moore [b], R.M. Merion [c], A.M.I. Azimzadeh [a]

[a] *University of Maryland Medical Center and Baltimore VAMC, Cardiac Surgery N4W94, 22 South Greene St., Baltimore, MD 21201, USA*

[b] *University Renal Research and Education Association, USA*

[c] *University of Michigan, MI, USA*

Abstract. ABO-incompatible lung transplantation has been described in four published cases, with two early deaths and two good long-term outcomes. Between 1992 and 2003, 41 additional cases have been reported to the US Scientific Registry of Transplant Recipients (SRTR). In these cases, only five early deaths (two directly ascribable to primary graft failure) have occurred, an overall incidence (12%) not significantly different than that observed for lung transplants between blood-type compatible individuals. This retrospective registry data suggest that the ABO barrier can be transgressed for the lung. Theoretical and experimental considerations relevant to transplantation in the context of preformed or induced anti-graft antibody are reviewed. © 2006 Published by Elsevier B.V.

Keywords: ABO-incompatible transplant; Lung transplant; Hyperacute rejection; Antibody-mediated rejection

1. Introduction

Lung transplantation is generally avoided in the context of ABO blood group incompatibility because of the presumption that hyperacute rejection or accelerated humoral injury (vascular rejection) will be caused by preformed antibody reactive with antigens expressed on donor endothelium [1–4]. The lung's response to immune injury mediated by antibody reactive with graft antigens is well established. Preformed and elicited antibodies are associated with acute lung injury in allograft [5] and xenograft models [6]. Antibody is also found in association with chronic rejection in animal models [7] and in man, where the antibody may be directed at HLA molecules [8,9] or against

* Corresponding author. Tel.: +1 11 410 328 5842; fax: +1 11 410 328 2750.
E-mail address: rpierson@smail.umaryland.edu (R.N. Pierson).

0531-5131/ © 2006 Published by Elsevier B.V.
doi:10.1016/j.ics.2006.03.052

non-HLA epithelial or endothelial antigens [10,11]. Experimental and clinical experience thus supports the plausible thesis that antibody reactive with antigens expressed by the graft is mechanistically linked to lung allograft dysfunction.

2. Clinical experience

2.1. Case reports

Only two cases of ABO-incompatible lung transplantation have been reported in the peer-reviewed literature. Updated clinical information regarding these patients was obtained by contact with primary physicians. Two additional experiences reported only in the lay press are briefly discussed based on published reports.

In 2002, we reported on management of an ABO blood group B patient who received a blood group A1 left single lung transplant in the context of a low anti-A antibody titer (1:4 by hemagglutination) [12]. Rising anti-A antibody during the second week was managed using antigen-specific immunoadsorption against A_{tri}-PAA-Sepharose, complement inhibition with recombinant soluble complement receptor type 1 (TP 10) and anti-CD20. The patient developed evidence of both graft accommodation and antigen-specific immunomodulation, and lived for over 4 years before succumbing to acute-on-chronic respiratory insufficiency and multisystem organ failure of uncertain pathogenesis. Banner et al. reported a successful outcome after inadvertent ABO-incompatible lung transplant [13]. An A-to-O bilateral lung recipient with a high anti-A titer (1:256) was treated with intraoperative plasmapheresis followed by non-antigen-specific immunoadsorption, IVIg and anti-CD20. Early graft dysfunction was not seen, anti-A antibody titers remained low and the patient was clinically well beyond 3 years. These experiences support the registry findings (reviewed below) that ABO-incompatible lung allografting can be associated with good outcomes, as for kidney, liver, heart and bone marrow (reviewed elsewhere in this volume).

In contrast, two cases have been reported recently in the lay press where ABO mismatched lung transplantation was performed inadvertently with poor outcomes. In 2003, a 66-year-old Israeli died shortly after receiving a single lung transplant of "the wrong blood type" [14]. Earlier that year a heart–lung block from a blood type A donor was transplanted into a blood-type O recipient [15,16]. Although the initial clinical course was unremarkable, ventilator support was never withdrawn and the recipient's respiratory function deteriorated toward the end of the first week for uncertain reasons; a blood type-compatible heart–lung block was implanted, but irreversible neurologic injury led to withdrawal of support. The role of anti-ABO antibody in lung injury and patient demise in these cases cannot be ascertained based on the information available.

2.2. US registry data

In September 2005, the US Organ Procurement and Transplant Network (OPTN) database was queried for instances of ABO-incompatible lung transplantation between 1/1/92 and 12/31/03. Identified cases were tabulated by category of ABO mismatch, with median survival duration reported for each category of cause of death. Forty-two patients received ABO-incompatible lung allografts during the study interval, representing 0.4% of 9804 first-time lung allografts (Table 1). Surprisingly, only two instances of death due to

Table 1
Characteristics and outcomes of 42 ABO-incompatible lung transplants (1992–2003)

Mismatch		Alive (2005)	Deaths early (<60 days)	<1 year	>1 year
A to B	1	0			1
A1 to O	27	12	1	3	11
A2 to O	2	0	1[a]		1
AB to O	3	2			1
AB to A	4	0			4
B to A	2	0	2[a]		
B to O	3	0	1		2
Summary	42	14	5 (12%)	3	20

[a] Early deaths ascribed to causes other than primary graft failure.

graft failure within the first year were reported, both occurring 3 days after transplant. Three other patients died within 60 days, two with bacterial septicemia at 10 and 56 days, and one of bronchial dehiscence at 4 days. Respiratory failure was reported as the cause of death in two of three additional cases, occurring at 93 and 442 days after transplant. Whether graft dysfunction attributable to anti-ABO antibody caused or contributed to any of these five early (<60 days) or three intermediate-term (<1 year) deaths cannot be ascertained from the registry data. A patient-specific audit of the registry data to further investigate this unexpected finding would be desirable. Overall reported 60-day (12%) and 1-year (19%) mortality for ABO-incompatible lung transplantation is similar to overall lung transplant outcomes [17].

Between 1992 and 2003, hyperacute rejection was reported as the cause of death in 29 patients (0.6% of deaths reported to SRTR) (Table 2). Among these 29 patients, the median time to death was 9 days and the average was about 3 months. Antibody against HLA antigens was detected in a minority of patients dying of hyperacute lung rejection: PRA $\geq$ 10% was detected in sera from only 35% (current) to 45% (peak historical) of these patients. None of the 42 ABO mismatched patients were also identified in response to the HAR query, suggesting that the risk of hyperacute rejection in this context is low.

These data and related conclusion must be considered in the context of several very important caveats. Data entry errors in recording donor or recipient ABO blood type could falsely increase the number of reported ABO mismatched lung transplants. An audit will require IRB approvals, and raises concerns about patient confidentiality and potential liability and adverse publicity for involved programs. In clinical practice, it is difficult to

Table 2
PRA titer, 29 lung recipients with HALR, 1992–2003

	Most recent before transplant	Peak historical
PRA “titer”	*N*	N
0.0	15	13
<10%	4	3
10–40%	4	5
>40%	4	5
Not available	2	3

reliably distinguish primary graft failure (which occurs in up to 15% of lung transplant recipients) from hyperacute lung rejection (HALR), particularly in the absence of anti-donor antibody, and thus it is possible that HALR is underreported. On the other hand, attribution of graft failure to HALR after the first days following transplant is implausible and indicates that unconventional definitions are being used in clinical practice. Inaccurate category assignment is an important confounding variable in any registry study and difficult to systematically audit or correct.

3. Antibody-induced lung injury: theoretical and experimental considerations

Abundant evidence indicates that the lung is particularly susceptible to injury by humoral mechanisms [6]. In addition to antibody and complement, cytokines, eicosanoids and coagulation cascade byproducts are humoral factors that have each been implicated in the pathogenesis of acute lung injury. Based on work in xenograft and other models, healthy endothelium with intact complement regulatory and anticoagulant function is resistant to injury by low titers of alloantibody or antibody to carbohydrate ABO antigens, but can be overwhelmed by higher titers, or by activation of or injury to endothelium. Endothelial vulnerability may be caused primarily by loss of defensive membrane proteins induced with endothelial activation in association with brain death and ischemia/reperfusion (I/R) injury.

Multiple cellular mechanisms also participate in acute lung injury, both through adhesion of platelets and blood leukocytes to areas of lung injury, and through the action of cells resident within the lung. As a consequence, the lung is particularly susceptible to dysfunction from the inflammatory response triggered by these cells. Alveolar, interstitial and intravascular macrophages express inflammatory mediators within minutes after exposure to LPS, and are primed by TNF and other cytokines to trigger a proinflammatory and procoagulant cascade of molecular and cellular events [18–21]. These immunocytes are anatomically stationed so as to rapidly and efficiently recruit neutrophils and other immune defense mechanisms to areas where "danger" is first encountered [22]. Macrophages participate in endotoxin-induced ALI in rodents and pigs [23,24], as do other monocytes, granulocytes (eosinophils, basophils and neutrophils) and platelets. Multiple cytokines and other inflammatory mediators elaborated by these cells promote endothelial activation and coagulation cascade activation. Blood monocytes and platelets traversing the lung then adhere to and interact with activated lung endothelium [6]. Reciprocal activating events in these cell populations trigger elaboration of tissue-factor-expressing microparticles, which then trigger local (and systemic) coagulation pathway activation, inflammation and thrombosis.

The variety of different mechanisms and mediators considered here illustrate the complexity of preventing lung injury. As a solution, current efforts hope to identify the convergence of multiple pathways on a prototypic tissue response phenotype, presumably mediated by common cell surface receptors and primitive intracellular proinflammatory cascades [25–29]. If so, induction of anti-apoptotic or anti-inflammatory gene cassettes may prove a practical approach to abort these responses. Pharmacologic manipulations of cAMP-dependent cytoprotective mechanisms may also prove useful to prevent or reverse acute lung injury mediated by antibody or other immune and non-immune mechanisms [30].

Three recent clinical reports suggests that humoral injury to the lung can occur relatively late after transplant (weeks to months) in the absence of demonstrable antibody responses to donor histocompatibility antigens [10,11,31,32]. Most survivors were treated with intensification of immunosuppressive therapy and some with plasmapheresis. All four reports speculate that this phenomenon represents a form of antibody-mediated acute vascular rejection, but its pathogenesis remains uncertain because immunohistologic and serologic information from these cases is incomplete.

Conventionally defined alloantibody directed at human lymphocyte-associated (HLA) antigens has a well-demonstrated role in acute and chronic lung injury. Hyperacute lung rejection associated with documented donor-reactive antibody has been reported in four cases, with mortality in three of four. Similar effects may be expected with ABO-incompatible lung allografts, particularly in the context of a high or rising antibody titer. Patients with detectable alloantibody are at increased risk for chronic rejection, whether or not the antibody cross-reacts with donor lymphocytes or other "irrelevant" HLA antigens. Those with high titers are at particularly high risk of poor long-term survival, suggesting that this is a marker for increased immune reactivity. Although the tissue distribution, density and linkage to cell signaling pathways differ significantly between HLA and ABO antigens, high titer responses to either class of antigens is likely to have adverse consequences for graft function. Whether low titers of antibody or antibody of particular isotypes promote or sustain accommodation remains conjectural.

Very limited data have been published on preventive strategies to protect lung allografts in the context of planned transplant across a positive cross-match. Two highly sensitized patients awaiting lung transplantation and four similar heart candidates were treated immediately preceding transplantation included 1–1.5 volume plasmapheresis, replacement with albumin and FFP, and infusion of ≥ 15 g high-dose intravenous immunoglobulin [33]. PRA reduction was generally incomplete and cross-matches remained positive at transplant, but graft dysfunction was not observed in the two lung allograft recipients, who died of CMV (7 months) and obliterative bronchiolitis (>4 years). The Harefield case, where ABO-incompatible graft injury was not seen despite an anti-A titer of 1:256 [13], and a Minnesota case [34], where anti-HLA A2-associated HAR was apparently reversed, indicate that immediate plasmapheresis with selective or non-selective reduction in titer of pathogenic antibodies is a rational approach to prevent humoral graft injury in this circumstance. These cases and our Vanderbilt experience indicate that accommodation and antigen-specific tolerance can occur, although the conditions required to accomplish this remain uncertain.

4. Summary: prospects for ABO-incompatible lung transplantation

In the only two cases documented in the peer-reviewed literature and based on registry review, ABO-incompatible lung transplant is associated with excellent short and intermediate results, without clinical evidence of humoral injury to the graft and late evidence of "accommodation" between the patient and the graft.

These favorable outcomes must be viewed with caution in light of two other incompletely documented adverse outcomes reported in the lay press, and inferior intermediate- and long-term outcomes associated with preformed or induced antibodies to

HLA antigens in lung and other organ allograft recipients. Although hyperacute lung rejection has been successfully managed on one reported case [34] and ECMO could offer a strategy to bridge to organ recovery (as shown for ischemia/reperfusion injury) [35], substantially increased mortality and impaired lung function should be expected unless steps are taken to actively diminish a high ABO titer and/or inhibit complement activation prior to graft perfusion. In our judgment, an ELISA assay specific for the donor ABO antigen, antigen-specific immunoadsorption and judicious use of an anti-complement agent represent the safest, most selective approaches to optimally diagnose induction of antigraft antibody and protect an ABO-mismatched lung allograft from injury during the critical period (speculatively, 30–45 days) before accommodation occurs. Anti-CD20 and anti-T-cell therapy were used in both successful ABO-incompatible cases, but whether they are necessary is unknown. In summary, ABO-mismatched lung allografting should be undertaken electively only after deliberate consideration of alternatives, and for appropriately informed recipients who are sufficiently robust to withstand the substantial additional physiologic stress associated with pheresis, supplemental immunosuppressive interventions, and their inevitable associated complications.

References

[1] T.E. Starzl, et al., Renal homografts in patients with major donor–recipient blood group incompatibilities, Surgery 55 (1964) 195–200.
[2] J. Dausset, F.T. Rapaport, The role of blood group antigens in human histocompatibility, Ann. N.Y. Acad. Sci. 129 (1966) 408.
[3] P.I. Terasaki, ABO mismatching errors in heart transplants, Lancet 362 (9380) (2003) 332.
[4] D.J. Cook, B. Graver, P.I. Terasaki, ABO incompatibility in cadaver donor kidney allografts, Transplant. Proc. 19 (6) (1987) 4549–4552.
[5] M. Yamane, Y. Sano, N. Shimizu, Significant changes in the alloantibody after lung transplantation in the cyclosporine treated rat model, Transplant. Immunol. 12 (2) (2004) 143–150.
[6] B.N. Nguyen, A.M. Azimzadeh, R.N. Pierson III, Beyond antibody-mediated rejection: hyperacute lung rejection as a paradigm for dysregulated inflammation, Curr. Drug Targets: Cardiovasc. Hematol. Disord. 5 (3) (2005) 255–269.
[7] J.S. Allan, et al., Modeling chronic lung allograft rejection in miniature swine, Transplantation 73 (3) (2002) 447–453.
[8] D. Hadjiliadis, et al., Pre-transplant panel reactive antibody in lung transplant recipients is associated with significantly worse post-transplant survival in a multicenter study, J. Heart Lung Transplant. 24 (7) (2005) S249–S254.
[9] J.D. Smith, et al., The effect of panel reactive antibodies and the donor specific crossmatch on graft survival after heart and heart–lung transplantation, Transplant. Immunol. 1 (1) (1993) 60–65.
[10] C.M. Magro, et al., Evidence that humoral allograft rejection in lung transplant patients is not histocompatibility antigen-related, Am. J. Transp. 3 (10) (2003) 1264–1272.
[11] A. Jaramillo, et al., Immune mechanisms in the pathogenesis of bronchiolitis obliterans syndrome after lung transplantation, Pediatr. Transplant. 9 (1) (2005) 84–93.
[12] R.N. Pierson III, et al., Successful management of an ABO-mismatched lung allograft using antigen-specific immunoadsorption, complement inhibition, and immunomodulatory therapy, Transplantation 74 (1) (2002) 79–84.
[13] N.R. Banner, et al., Management of an ABO-incompatible lung transplant, Am. J. Transp. 4 (7) (2004 Jul) 1192–1196.
[14] Transplant News, 2004 (March 9), p. 7.
[15] D. Resnick, The Jesica Santillan tragedy: lessons learned, Hastings Cent. Rep. 33 (4) (2003 Jul–Aug) 15–20.

[16] E.W. Campion, A death at Duke, N. Engl. J. Med. 348 (12) (2003 Mar 20) 1083–1084.
[17] R.N. Pierson III, et al., Thoracic organ transplantation, Am. J. Transp. 4 (Suppl. 9) (2004) 93–105.
[18] T.S. Maxey, et al., Tumor necrosis factor-alpha from resident lung cells is a key initiating factor in pulmonary ischemia–reperfusion injury, J. Thorac. Cardiovasc. Surg. 127 (2) (2004) 541–547.
[19] C.G. Chitko-McKown, et al., Porcine alveolar and pulmonary intravascular macrophages: comparison of immune functions, J. Leukoc. Biol. 50 (4) (1991) 364–372.
[20] B.J. Collins, et al., Thromboxane mediates pulmonary hypertension and lung inflammation during hyperacute lung rejection, J. Appl. Physiol. 90 (6) (2001) 2257–2268.
[21] J.T. Berg, et al., Depletion of alveolar macrophages by liposome-encapsulated dichloromethylene diphosphonate, J. Appl. Physiol. 74 (6) (1993) 2812–2819.
[22] P. Matzinger, The danger model: a renewed sense of self, Science 296 (5566) (2002) 301–305.
[23] M.B. Everhart, et al., Intratracheal administration of liposomal clodronate accelerates alveolar macrophage reconstitution following fetal liver transplantation, J. Leukoc. Biol. 77 (2) (2005) 173–180.
[24] J.G. Gaca, et al., Prevention of acute lung injury in swine: depletion of pulmonary intravascular macrophages using liposomal clodronate, J. Surg. Res. 112 (1) (2003) 19–25.
[25] M.S. Mulligan, et al., Protective effects of oligosaccharides in P-selectin-dependent lung injury, Nature 364 (6433) (1993) 149–151.
[26] M.S. Mulligan, et al., C5a-dependent up-regulation in vivo of lung vascular P-selectin, J. Immunol. 158 (4) (1997) 1857–1861.
[27] J.A. Nick, et al., Recombinant human activated protein C reduces human endotoxin-induced pulmonary inflammation via inhibition of neutrophil chemotaxis, Blood 104 (13) (2004) 3878–3885.
[28] B.J. McVerry, J.G.N. Garcia, Endothelial cell barrier regulation by sphingosine 1-phosphate, J. Cell. Biochem. 92 (2004) 1075–1085.
[29] J.H. Finigan, et al., Activated protein C mediates novel lung endothelial barrier enhancement: role of sphingosine 1-phosphate receptor transactivation, J. Biol. Chem. (2005).
[30] P.L. Khimenko, et al., Adenosine A2 receptors reverse ischemia–reperfusion lung injury independent of beta-receptors, J. Appl. Physiol. 78 (3) (1995) 990–996.
[31] D.B. Badesch, et al., Pulmonary capillaritis: a possible histologic form of acute pulmonary allograft rejection, J. Heart Lung Transplant. 17 (4) (1998) 415–422.
[32] G.G. Miller, et al., Acute humoral rejection of human lung allografts and elevation of C4d in bronchoalveolar lavage fluid, Am. J. Transp. 4 (8) (2004) 1323–1330.
[33] J.A. Robinson, et al., Plasmapheresis followed by intravenous immunoglobulin in presensitized patients awaiting thoracic organ transplantation, Ther. Apher. 1 (2) (1997) 147–151.
[34] H.B. Bittner, et al., Hyperacute rejection in single lung transplantation-case report of successful management by means of plasmapheresis and antithymocyte globulin treatment, Transplantation 71 (5) (2001) 649–651.
[35] P.S. Dahlberg, et al., Medium-term results of extracorporeal membrane oxygenation for severe acute lung injury after lung transplantation, J. Heart Lung Transplant. 23 (2004) 979–984.

Memorial lecture

International Congress Series 1292 (2006) 73–87

www.ics-elsevier.com

A new immunosuppressive therapy in ABO-incompatible kidney transplantation based on a new concept of accommodation

Kota Takahashi*

Division of Urology, Department of Regenerative and Transplant Medicine, Graduate School of Medical and Dental Sciences, Niigata University, Asahimachi 1, Niigata 951-8510, Niigata, Japan

Abstract. Since the advent of modern immunology, there have been two major principles in transplantation medicine: tolerance and accommodation. Owing to the shortage of cadaveric kidneys in Japan, since 1989, we have performed ABO-incompatible kidney transplantation to expand the indication for kidney transplantation. Through our experience, we have studied the basic and clinical characteristics of accommodation. During the past half-century, we were taught that ABO-incompatible kidney transplantation would result in hyperacute rejection and graft loss within 24 h after transplantation. However, rejection does not occur and the grafts survived in nearly all recipients of ABO-incompatible kidney transplants. We found that accommodation is the mysterious phenomenon responsible for graft survival despite the presence of ABO antigens on graft endothelial cells and of antibodies to these antigens in the recipient's blood. We initially thought that ABO antigens and HLA antigens could not be changed or modified. However, our experience with ABO-incompatible kidney transplantation shows that these two types of antigens differ. ABO antigens are governed by the ABO gene product ABO glycosyltransferase. ABO antigens cannot express antigenicity in the absence of this enzyme. During accommodation, the recipient's ABO genes suppress ABO genes in the graft, thereby inhibiting production of ABO glycosyltransferase. Antigenicity of graft ABO antigens is thus lost, leading to graft survival. Immunosuppressive therapy has been established on the basis of the theory of accommodation. In Japan, ABO-incompatible kidney transplantation has been performed in >700 patients. Outcomes are similar to those of ABO-compatible kidney transplantation. Throughout the world including Europe and North America, ABO-incompatible kidney transplantation has been evaluated as safe and effective as ABO-compatible transplantation and is now applied for all types of organ transplantation. Since the discovery of human ABO blood type by Karl Landsteiner in 1901, 100 years were required to break through the wall of ABO blood type, a dream of transplantation medicine. We have delineated the

* Tel.: +81 25 227 2284; fax: +81 25 227 0784.
E-mail address: kota@med.niigata-u.ac.jp.

doi:10.1016/j.ics.2006.03.054

mechanism of accommodation, leading to the establishment of new strategies for immunosuppressive therapy and enabling ABO-incompatible kidney transplantation to be performed throughout the world. We believe that this represents a major advance in transplantation medicine.

Keywords: ABO-incompatibility; Accommodation; Hyperacute rejection; Antibody-mediated rejection; Immunosuppression; Kidney transplantation; Splenectomy

1. Introduction

Outcomes of ABO-incompatible kidney transplantation have dramatically improved since the discovery of the mechanism of accommodation and development of immunosuppressive therapy based on accommodation. Herein are reported recent findings on accommodation and new therapeutic strategies for ABO-incompatible kidney transplantation developed on the basis of accommodation [1–5]. Current knowledge about ABO-incompatible kidney transplantation is reviewed.

2. New findings obtained by performing ABO-incompatible kidney transplantation

(1) The presence of the ABO gene product ABO glycosyltransferase plays an extremely important role in ABO-incompatible kidney transplantation.
(2) ABO antigens differ from HLA antigens. It was previously thought that ABO antigens and HLA antigens could not be changed, but ABO-incompatible kidney transplantation has shown that these two types of antigens differ. ABO antigens are governed by ABO glycosyltransferase; their antigenicity thus depends on this enzyme.
(3) It was originally thought that hyperacute rejection would occur within 24 h after ABO-incompatible kidney transplantation. Conversely, however, ABO-related hyperacute rejection does not occur. We have previously reported the reasons for this observation.
(4) The mechanism of antibody-mediated rejection (delayed hyperacute rejection) occurring 2–7 days after transplantation has been reported.
(5) The mechanism responsible for graft survival in ABO-incompatible kidney transplantation (i.e., the mechanism of accommodation) can now be explained.

ABO glycosyltransferase, linking the ABO blood type gene to ABO antigens, has been shown to play a key role in these phenomena [3–5].

3. Outcomes of ABO-incompatible kidney transplantation in Japan

Through all of our efforts, outcomes of ABO-incompatible kidney transplantation in Japan have significantly improved since 2001, when rates of graft survival reached 96% and 94% at 1 and 3 years, respectively. Graft survival rates have significantly improved by 14 percentage points at 1 year and by 13 percentage points at 3 years as compared with those for 1989 through 1991. These improvements are mainly attributed

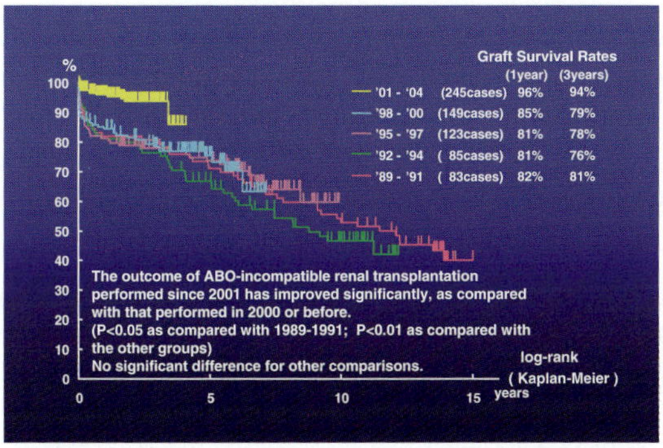

Fig. 1. Graft-survival rates after ABO-incompatible kidney transplantation according to year in Japan. The outcome of ABO-incompatible kidney transplantation performed since 2001 was significantly better than that performed in 2000 or previously.

to the decreased mortality and lower incidence of acute antibody-mediated rejection (Fig. 1).

4. Reasons for performing ABO-incompatible kidney transplantation

My involvement with ABO-incompatible kidney transplantation started with the care of children with chronic renal failure. In the 1980s, the level of medical care for children with chronic renal failure remained extremely poor, despite the efforts of many pediatricians and researchers. Hemodialysis and kidney transplantation were effective treatments for end-stage renal failure; however, hemodialysis adversely affected growth and development of children and caused complications such as severe renal rickets. Kidney transplantation was therefore necessary for cure.

Questionnaire surveys conducted by the Japanese Society for Pediatric Nephrology in the 1980s indicated that incompatibility of blood type between donor and recipient was the main reason for not performing kidney transplantation in children with end-stage renal failure, even if their parents had requested such treatment. ABO-incompatible kidney transplantation was expected to lead to hyperacute rejection with immediate graft loss within 24 h after transplantation. Even today, nearly all textbooks on transplantation medicine warn that ABO-incompatible kidney transplantation will result in hyperacute rejection with graft loss. We continued to be taught that this is true and considered hyperacute rejection an inevitable consequence of ABO-incompatible kidney transplantation.

5. Difficulties in performing ABO-incompatible kidney transplantation

My impression about the history of ABO-incompatible kidney transplantation can be summarized as “a struggle against partially incorrect, fixed concepts in immunology”. For example, we had to overcome the following types of incorrect concepts.

We first performed ABO-incompatible kidney transplantation in Japan on January 19, 1989. We were very concerned that hyperacute rejection would occur after transplantation, immediately leading to graft loss. Since then, we have performed ABO-incompatible kidney transplantation in about 150 patients. Each time we performed ABO-incompatible kidney transplantation, we questioned why hyperacute rejection leading to graft loss did not occur within 24 h after transplantation in even one patient.

6. Timing of antibody-mediated rejection after ABO-incompatible kidney transplantation

Statistical data on ABO-incompatible kidney transplantation in Japan have been compiled since 1997. After ABO-incompatible kidney transplantation had been performed in about 400 patients, we surveyed the most common times for antibody-mediated rejection to occur after transplantation. Surprisingly, hyperacute rejection did not spontaneously occur within 24 h after transplantation in any patient. Nearly all cases of antibody-mediated rejection occurred between 2 and 7 days after transplantation [3–5].

7. Comparison of outcomes of ABO-incompatible with ABO-compatible kidney transplantation

In 1989, the year we started to perform ABO-incompatible kidney transplantation, we were concerned that ABO antigens on endothelial cells of transplanted kidney would be continuously exposed to anti-A and anti-B antibodies in the recipient's blood, thereby increasing risk of chronic allograft nephropathy (CAN). We had assumed that long-term outcome of ABO-incompatible kidney transplantation would be worse than that of ABO-compatible kidney transplantation. In contrast to our expectations, however, with currently available immunosuppressive therapy, we found that long-term outcomes did not significantly differ between ABO-incompatible and ABO-compatible kidney transplantation. This finding suggests that induction and establishment of accommodation occur relatively early after transplantation (Fig. 2) [2–6].

8. Accommodation, a mysterious phenomenon

Accommodation is a very mysterious phenomenon. Despite the presence of ABO antigens on endothelial cells of the graft and of anti-A and anti-B antibodies in the

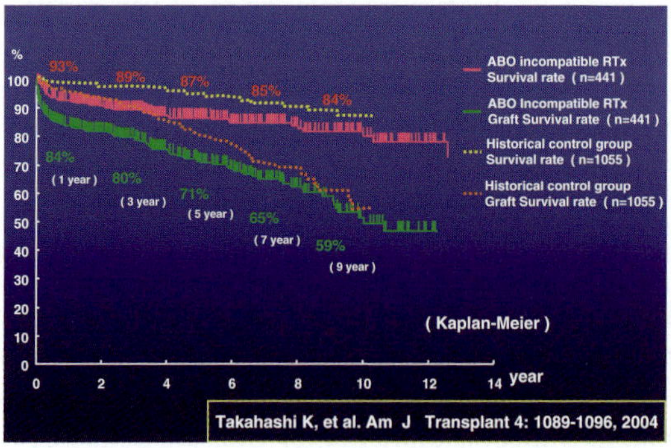

Fig. 2. Patient survival rate and graft survival rate in recipients of ABO-incompatible kidney transplants and historical control group in Japan.

recipient's blood, ABO-antigen-antibody reaction does not occur. This phenomenon is referred to as accommodation [2–5]. Why does it occur?

Severe delayed hyperacute rejection can rarely occur between 2 and 7 days after transplantation. Accommodation is induced about 1–2 weeks after transplantation. Once established, accommodation continues as long as the graft survives. These findings led to the discovery of the mechanism of accommodation, i.e., that responsible for graft survival in ABO-incompatible kidney transplantation [2–5].

9. Differences between ABO and HLA antigens

Since the advent of modern immunology, we believed that ABO and HLA antigens could not be changed or modified. However, our experience with ABO-incompatible kidney transplantation showed that these two types of antigens differ. ABO antigens are governed by ABO glycosyltransferase (ABO genes–ABO glycosyltransferase–ABO antigens). ABO antigens cannot express their antigenicity in the absence of glycosyltransferase.

In contrast, HLA antigens, markers that enable identification of donor and recipient cells, are directly governed by genes of the HLA complex (HLA genes–HLA antigens). Therefore, these genes and their antigenicity cannot be changed. ABO glycosyltransferase is thus implicated in the mechanism underlying graft survival in ABO-incompatible kidney transplantation (i.e., accommodation), the mechanism by which hyperacute rejection does not occur, and the mechanism by which acute antibody-mediated rejection rarely develops between 2 and 7 days after transplantation [3–5].

10. Why does hyperacute rejection not occur in ABO-incompatible kidney transplantation?

Donor kidneys are preserved by ice cooling. Enzymes such as ABO glycosyltransferase require conditions of 36–37 °C for activation and are permanently inactivated at lower temperatures. Antigens on blood vessels also lose their antigenicity and these inactivated antigens do not react with ABO antibodies in the recipient's blood. Thus, hyperacute rejection does not occur (Fig. 3) [3–5].

11. Onset of delayed hyperacute rejection and induction and establishment of accommodation

The reason for the rare occurrence of very severe delayed hyperacute rejection between 2 and 7 days after transplantation has been reported [3,4]. Around this time, after resumption of blood flow, endothelial cells undergo regeneration leading to production of ABO glycosyltransferase and return of antigenicity of ABO antigens. Severe rejection may occur at this time unless antibody production is inhibited by immunosuppressive therapy. Once severe rejection occurs, nearly all recipients exhibit graft loss.

With currently available immunosuppressive therapy, accommodation is induced in >90% of recipients of ABO-incompatible kidney transplants. About 1 week after transplantation, ABO genes in the recipient dominate and suppress those in the donor organ, thereby inhibiting production of ABO glycosyltransferase. Antigenicity of ABO

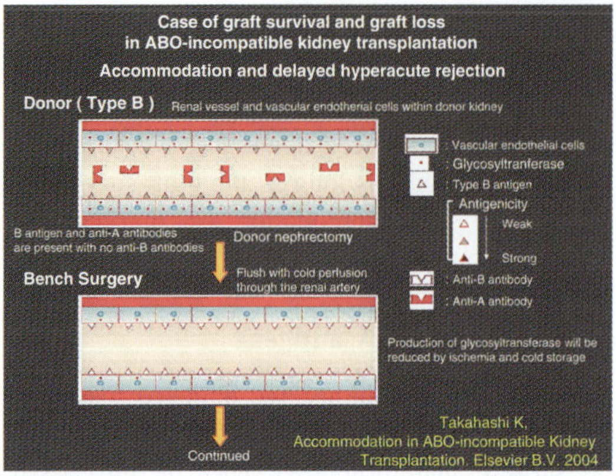

Fig. 3. ABO-incompatible kidney transplantation involving a donor with blood type B and a recipient with blood type O. The donor kidney was immediately preserved by ice cooling until the time of transplantation.

antigens of the donor organ is thus lost. In other words, accommodation is induced and the ABO-incompatible graft survives (Fig. 4) [3–5].

12. Changes of ABO glycosyltransferase in blood

As for changes of ABO glycosyltransferase, if the kidney from a blood type B donor is transplanted into a blood type O recipient B-type glycosyltransferase, originally not

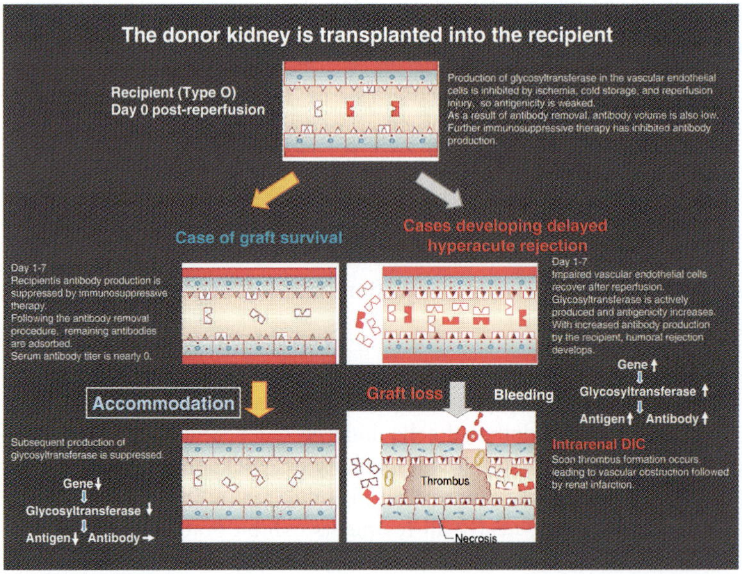

Fig. 4. In nearly all recipients of ABO-incompatible kidney transplants, accommodation was established and the graft survived (left panel). If the production of anti-A and anti-B antibodies by the recipient is not inhibited, delayed hyperacute rejection occurred between 2 and 7 days after transplantation (left panel).

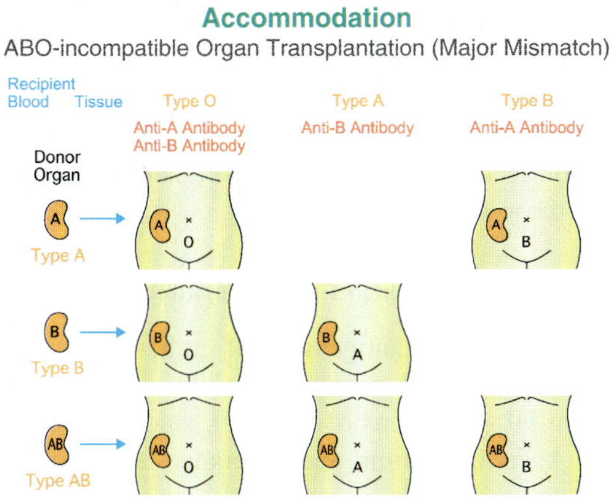

Fig. 5. Accommodation in successful ABO-incompatible solid-organ transplantation.

present in the recipient's blood, transiently appears in serum then gradually disappears [4,7].

13. Establishment of accommodation in ABO-incompatible organ transplantation and ABO minor-mismatch bone marrow transplantation

Fig. 5 shows possible combinations in ABO-incompatible organ transplantation. If the graft takes, accommodation is induced in all combinations. Accommodation also occurs in ABO minor-mismatch bone marrow transplantation.

Fig. 6 shows ABO blood types in donor (upper panel) and recipient (lower panel) in ABO minor-mismatch bone marrow transplantation. If the donor's bone marrow finally takes, the recipient's blood type changes into the donor's blood type. However, the blood type of the recipient's tissues remains unchanged. Despite the presence of antibodies in the

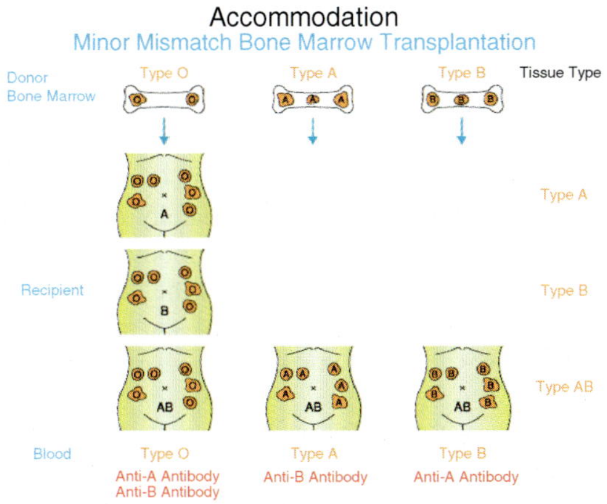

Fig. 6. Accommodation in successful ABO minor-mismatch bone marrow transplantation.

recipient's blood and of antigens in the recipient's tissue, nothing happens. This phenomenon suggests that accommodation is established.

In patients with surviving grafts after ABO-incompatible organ transplantation or ABO minor-mismatch bone marrow transplantation, accommodation has thus been established. Given the mechanism of accommodation, ABO genes derived from bone marrow may dominate and suppress those in tissue [5].

14. Differences between accommodation and tolerance

Accommodation refers to loss of antigenicity of graft ABO antigens resulting in graft survival. In contrast, tolerance is the process by which recipients' lymphocytes become unresponsive to different HLA antigens of the graft, since antigenicity of HLA antigens cannot be modified. Accommodation and tolerance are thus completely different phenomena.

15. Decrease of serum antibody titer after establishment of accommodation and causes thereof

In ABO-incompatible kidney transplantation, serum antibody titer after establishment of accommodation is lower than that before transplantation. Antibody titer is particularly low relative to the histo-blood type of the donor graft. In ABO minor-mismatch bone marrow transplantation, antibody titer relative to the histo-blood type of the recipient organ is zero.

How should we interpret these data? First, consumption of produced antibodies may result in low or zero antibody titers. If antibodies are consumed, antibody-mediated rejection or CAN might be expected to occur in recipients of ABO-incompatible kidney transplants. Consumption of antibodies would also probably lead to peripheral circulatory disturbances in recipients of ABO minor-mismatch bone marrow transplants. However, these phenomena do not occur following establishment of accommodation in such recipients.

The second most plausible reason for decreased antibody titer is inhibition of antibody production. A feedback system likely exists between blood type of the recipient and histo-type of the donor graft in ABO-incompatible kidney transplantation, as well as between blood type of donor bone marrow and histo-type of recipient in ABO minor-mismatch bone marrow transplantation.

Strictly speaking, to establish accommodation in ABO-incompatible kidney transplantation, the blood type of the recipient inhibits antigenicity of the histo-type of the donor graft and histo-type of the donor graft inhibits antibody production. In ABO minor-mismatch bone marrow transplantation, blood type of the donor graft inhibits antigenicity of the histo-type of the recipient and histo-type of the recipient suppresses antibody production. The author believes that this is the mechanism involved.

16. A new strategy for immunosuppressive therapy based on accommodation

Irrespective of the exact mechanism involved, it is currently acknowledged that accommodation is established in the recipient 1–2 weeks after transplantation if the clinical course is favorable during that period. Our studies have demonstrated that, once induced and established, accommodation continues as long as the graft survives.

On the basis of these observations, we have developed a new strategy for immunosuppressive therapy in which either ABO antigens or their antibodies are depleted during the approximately 1–2 weeks after transplantation, the period required for induction of accommodation. First, it is important extensively to remove anti-A and anti-B antibodies in serum before transplantation [8–10]. Secondly, adequate desensitization therapy should be started before transplantation to inhibit antibody production during the period before induction of accommodation [3–5,11].

17. Pinpoint-targeted immunosuppression

Fig. 7 shows examples of immunosuppressive therapy in ABO-incompatible kidney transplantation. Ideally, both T cell-and B cell-mediated immunity should be suppressed. However, once accommodation is established, ABO antigens of the graft lose their antigenicity. It is therefore sufficient to administer immunosuppressive therapy that suppresses mainly T cell-mediated immunity, similar to that used in ABO-compatible kidney transplantation (Fig. 7).

18. Clinical significance of splenectomy

We all know that the spleen produces antibodies. However, whether splenectomy is really required in ABO-incompatible transplantation is another matter. We previously performed splenectomy in all recipients of ABO-incompatible kidney transplants [2–5,11,12]. However, because we now know that accommodation is induced 1-2 weeks after transplantation we no longer regard splenectomy necessary to inhibit antibody production for only that period. Instead of splenectomy, adequate desensitization therapy should be started before transplantation to inhibit antibody production until accommodation is induced [3–5,11].

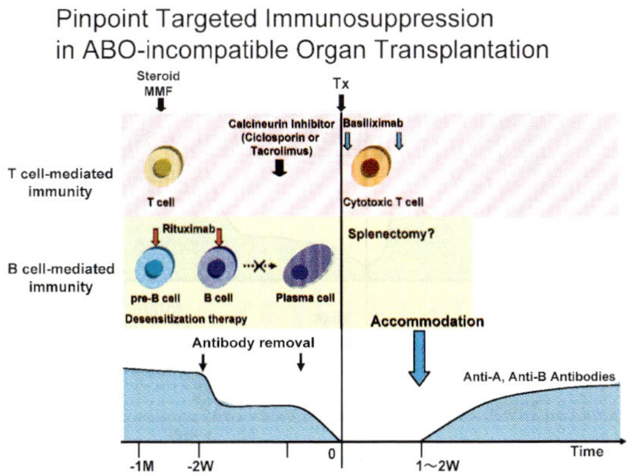

Fig. 7. Pinpoint-targeted immunosuppression in ABO-incompatible kidney transplantation.

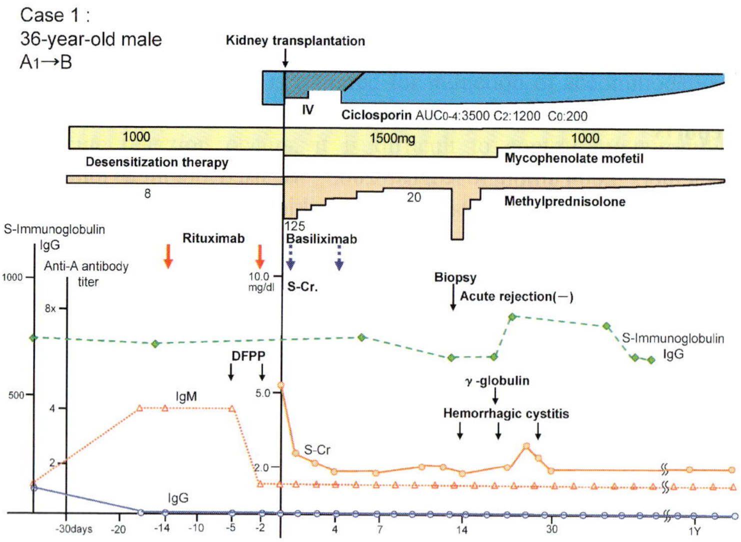

Fig. 9. Clinical course of patient 1.

Moreover, CD25 was completely inhibited by basiliximab, given during surgery and 4 days after transplantation. In contrast, pan-T cells CD3, CD4 and CD8 were nearly unchanged. We consequently refer to this immunosuppressive therapy as "pinpoint-targeted immunosuppression" (Fig. 10).

Patient 2 was a 66-year-old man with blood type A_1. The donor was his 60-year-old wife with blood type B. The patient received immunosuppressive therapy according to protocol. Immediately after transplantation, he developed atelectasis and aspiration pneumonia. Methicillin-resistant *Staphylococcus epidermidis* (MRSE) was isolated from both sputum and blood. Serum creatinine level dropped steadily to 3.4 mg/dl, but pneumonia did not improve. The transplanted kidney was therefore removed on day 9 after transplantation and immunosuppressive therapy withdrawn. He then responded to treatment with antibiotics and was discharged from hospital after 1 month.

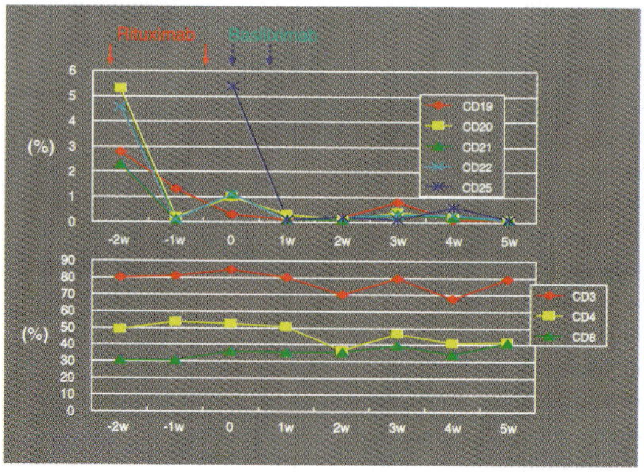

Fig. 10. Peripheral-blood lymphocyte subsets in patient 1.

Patient 3 was a 50-year-old man with blood type A_1. The donor was his 42-year-old wife with blood type A_1B. The patient received immunosuppressive therapy according to protocol. One week after transplantation, his serum creatinine level fell to 1.1 mg/dl. Two weeks after transplantation, the level increased. Biopsy of the transplanted kidney was therefore performed. The patient had acute cellular rejection of type IA according to the Banff classification and was therefore given methylprednisolone pulse therapy. Graft function recovered. Subsequently, the patient's condition steadily improved. As of 11 months after transplantation, serum creatinine was 1.1 mg/dl and urine negative for protein. During hospitalization, anti-B antibody titer was completely inhibited. As of 11 months after transplantation, anti-B antibody titer was 1:1.

22. New immunosuppressive therapy for ABO-incompatible kidney transplantation based on new concept of accommodation

B cell-mediated immunity was inhibited by desensitization therapy with mycophenolate mofetil and methylprednisolone given orally for 1 month before transplantation and rituximab given before operation. In addition, antibodies were removed by DFPP, thereby inhibiting antibody production until induction of accommodation.

To control T cell-mediated immunity, calcineurin inhibitor-based immunosuppressive therapy was given. Basiliximab was used to suppress activated T cells that did not respond to this regimen. Splenectomy was not required because antibody production was inhibited by desensitization therapy started 1 month before transplantation. Pinpoint-targeted immunosuppression is likely to become a standard regimen for immunosuppressive treatment in ABO-incompatible kidney transplantation.

These results show that ABO-incompatible kidney transplantation is as safe and effective as ABO-compatible kidney transplantation for the treatment of end-stage renal failure. More investigation is required further to improve outcomes of ABO-incompatible kidney transplantation.

23. Conclusion

Since the discovery of human ABO blood type by Karl Landsteiner in 1901, about 100 years were required to break through the wall of ABO blood type, a dream of transplantation medicine. In addition to overcoming this barrier, we have delineated the mechanism underlying graft survival, i.e., accommodation. These discoveries have led to establishment of new strategies for immunosuppressive therapy, enabling ABO-incompatible kidney transplantation to be performed throughout the world. We hope that our efforts will contribute to further advances in transplantation medicine [16–22].

Acknowledgements

The author wishes to express his gratitude for the continuing support and encouragement of everyone concerned. In addition, deep appreciation is expressed to Niigata University and Tokyo Women's Medical University for their invaluable help.

Definitions of terms

Accommodation: Absence of reaction between ABO blood group antigens on the surfaces of endothelial cells within the graft and the same antibodies in the recipient's blood, i.e., graft survival without antibody-mediated rejection [2–5].

Hyperacute rejection: Acute antibody-mediated rejection occurring within 24 h of transplantation.

Delayed hyperacute rejection: Antibody-mediated rejection occurring >24 h after transplantation [3–5].

References

[1] R.A. Montgomery, ABO incompatible transplantation: to B or not to B, Am. J. Transp. 4 (2004) 1011–1012.

[2] K. Takahashi, et al., Excellent long-term outcome of ABO-incompatible living donor kidney transplantation in Japan, Am. J. Transp. 4 (2004) 1089–1096.

[3] K. Takahashi, Accommodation in ABO-incompatible kidney transplantation: why do kidney grafts survive? Transplant. Proc. 36 (Suppl. 2S) (2004) 193–196.

[4] K. Takahashi, Accommodation, ABO-Incompatible Kidney Transplantation, Elsevier, Amsterdam, 2004, pp. 1–209.

[5] K. Takahashi, A new concept of accommodation in ABO-incompatible kidney transplantation, Clin. Transplant. 19 (Suppl. 14) (2005) 76–85.

[6] K. Takahashi, et al., First report of 7-year survey on ABO-incompatible kidney transplantation in Japan, Clin. Exp. Nephrol. 5 (2001) 119–125.

[7] K. Takahashi, ABO-Incompatible Kidney Transplantation, Elsevier, Amsterdam, 2001, pp. 1–159.

[8] H. Shimmura, et al., Role of anti-A/B antibody titers in results of ABO-incompatible kidney transplantation, Transplantation 70 (2000) 1331–1335.

[9] T. Agishi, et al., Immunoadsorption of anti-A or anti-B antibody for successful kidney transplantation between ABO incompatible pairs and its limitation, ASAIO Trans. 37 (1991) 496–498.

[10] H. Shimmura, et al., Removal of anti-A/B antibodies with plasmapheresis in ABO-incompatible kidney transplantation, Ther. Apheresis 4 (2000) 395–398.

[11] M. Manami, N. Mitsuhata, Improved outcomes after ABO-incompatible living-donor kidney transplantation after 4 weeks of treatment with mycophenolate mofetil, Transplantation 79 (2005) 1756–1758.

[12] G.P.J. Alexandre, et al., Human ABO incompatible living donor renal homografts, Neth. J. Med. 28 (1985) 231–234.

[13] G. Tyden, G. Kumlien, I. Fehrman, Successful ABO-incompatible kidney transplantations without splenectomy using antigen-specific immunoadsorption and rituximab, Transplantation 76 (2003) 730–743.

[14] J.M. Aranda, et al., Anti-CD20 monoclonal antibody (rituximab) therapy for acute cardiac humoral rejection: a case report, Transplantation 73 (2002) 907–910.

[15] T. Sawada, S. Fuchinoue, S. Teraoka, Successful A_1-to-O ABO-incompatible kidney transplantation after a preconditioning regimen consisting of anti-CD20 monoclonal antibody infusions, splenectomy, and double-filtration plasmapheresis, Transplantation 74 (2002) 1207–1210.

[16] D.S. Warren, et al., Successful renal transplantation across simultaneous ABO incompatible and positive crossmatch barriers, Am. J. Transp. 4 (2004) 561–568.

[17] D.W. Hanto, et al., ABO-incompatible liver transplantation with no immunological graft losses using total plasma exchange, splenectomy, and quadruple immunosuppression: evidence for accommodation, Liver Transplant. 9 (2003) 22–30.

[18] L.J. West, et al., ABO-incompatible heart transplantation in infants, N. Engl. J. Med. 344 (2001) 793–800.

[19] L. Rydberg, ABO-incompatibility in solid organ transplantation, Transfus. Med. 11 (2001) 325–342.

[20] P. Mohacsi, et al., Successful management of a B-type cardiac allograft into an O-type man with 3 1/2-year clinical follow-up, Transplantation 72 (2001) 1328–1330.
[21] R.N. Pierson III, et al., Successful management of an ABO-mismatched lung allograft using antigen-specific immunoadsorption, complement inhibition, and immunomodulatory therapy, Transplantation 74 (2002) 79–84.
[22] K. Takahashi, et al.for the Japanese Tacrolimus Study Group, Successful results after 5 years of tacrolimus therapy in ABO-incompatible kidney transplantation in Japan, Transplant. Proc. 37 (2005) 1800–1803.

Antibody removal

International Congress Series 1292 (2006) 91–95

www.ics-elsevier.com

The safety measures for double filtration plasma apheresis (DFPP) before ABO-incompatible kidney transplantation

S. Nishi [a,*], S. Hasegawa [a], F. Gejyo [a], K. Saito [b], Y. Nakagawa [b], K. Takahashi [b]

[a] *Blood Purification Center, Niigata University Medical and Dental Hospital, Japan*
[b] *Division of Urology, Graduate School of Medical and Dental Sciences, Niigata University, Japan*

Abstract. Double filtration plasma apheresis (DFPP) is an essential procedure for the success of ABO-incompatibility kidney transplantation. During DFPP treatment serum albumin fraction decreases as well as serum globulin fraction, therefore the drop of colloidal oncotic pressure induces intravascular dehydration. We raised the concentration of albumin solution as supplementation fluid from 7.5% to 12.5%. In DFPP treatment with 7.5% albumin supplementation solution, the reduction rate of serum albumin concentration, pre-albumin/post-albumin, was 0.821 ($p<0.05$, $n=8$), however, in DFPP treatment with 12.5% albumin supplementation solution, the rate of change of serum albumin concentration was 1.054 ($p=\text{ns}$, $n=7$). This insignificant change of serum albumin concentration resulted in the prevention of hypotension and other complications associated with intravascular dehydration derived from the drop of oncotic pressure due to DFPP treatment. Twelve and a half percent albumin solution as supplementation fluid is recommended for DFPP treatment before ABO-incompatible kidney transplantation.

Keywords: Double filtration plasma apheresis (DFPP); Oncotic pressure; Intravascular dehydration; Hypotension

1. Introduction

Antibody removal treatment is essential for the success of ABO-incompatible kidney transplantation. Among three procedures, plasma exchange, double filtration plasma apheresis (DFPP), and hemoadsorption, we have chosen DFPP, because of the

* Corresponding author. Tel.: +81 25 227 2770; fax: +81 25 227 0775.
E-mail address: snishi@med.niigata-u.ac.jp (S. Nishi).

0531-5131/
doi:10.1016/j.ics.2006.03.059

avoidance of viral sources contaminated in fresh frozen plasma (FFP) through the quarantine inspection [1–3] and the discontinuation of commercial supply of adsorption column. In DFPP, the modulation of albumin solution as supplementation fluid is extremely important from the viewpoint of the safety and efficacy performance.

Until now, albumin concentration as supplementation fluid was determined empirically in the each institution [4]. In our country from 7% to 8% albumin solution that was akin to the concentration of serum total protein has been normally used for DFPP treatment. In this condition, we could not often prevent the complications derived from the intravascular dehydration during DFPP treatment. In order to avoid the intravascular dehydration, we raised the concentration of albumin solution from 7.5% to 12.5% in our institution and evaluated the safety of this alteration in the recipients before ABO-incompatible kidney transplantation. This change dramatically reduced the adverse effects derived from the intravascular dehydration due to DFPP treatment.

2. Our data

Nine hemodialysis patients waiting for ABO-incompatible kidney transplantation were subjective. To all patients we explained the purpose of this research and received the consent from them. We followed the spirits of Declaration of Helsinki. DFPP was performed eight times with 7.5% albumin solution as supplementation fluid in 4 patients. Seven times were done with 12.5% albumin solution as supplementation fluid in 5 patients. In each DFPP we prepared 500-ml albumin solution as supplementation fluid. DFPP was performed on the day between dialysis treatments. DFPP treatment using OP-05 (plasma separator, Asahi Co.) and Cascadeflo EC-30W (second filter, Asahi Co.) was operated until the complete consumption of 500-ml supplementation fluid.

We measured the following serum markers; total protein, serum albumin, IgG and IgM, before and after DFPP. Blood pressure was monitored carefully from the start of DFPP and 24 h after the end of DFPP. We continuously evaluated the alteration of the blood volume by an optic continuous hematocrit monitor (Crit-line II, JMS Co.) that was attached in the circuit of DFPP.

As statistical method we used non-paired Student's t-test. The p value less than 0.05 was considered significant.

Fig. 1 reveals the mean levels of serum total protein and albumin before and after DFPP with 7.5% albumin solution as supplementation fluid in 8 DFPPs of 4 patients.

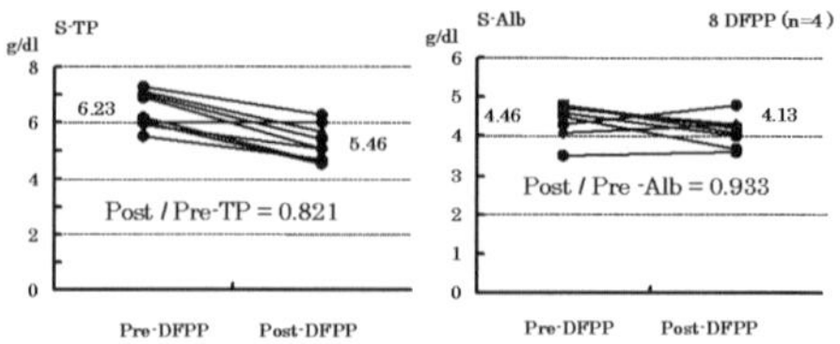

Fig. 1. Serum total protein and albumin concentrations before and after DFPP treatment with supplementation fluid of 7.5% albumin solution.

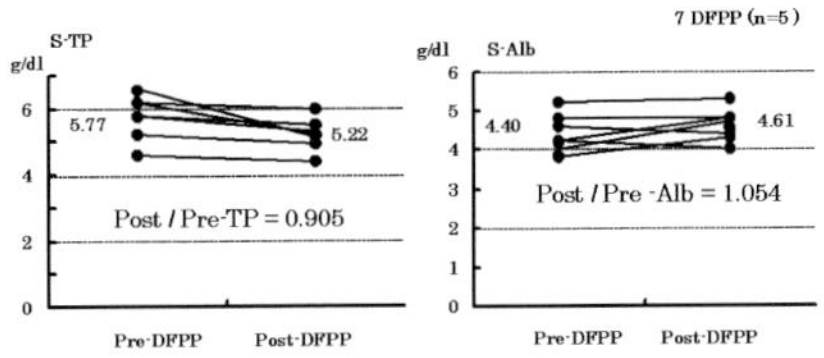

Fig. 2. Serum total protein and albumin concentrations before and after DFPP treatment with supplementation fluid of 12.5% albumin solution.

The mean serum total protein dropped significantly from 6.23 to 5.46 g/dl ($p<0.05$) and the mean serum albumin also fell significantly from 4.46 to 4.13 g/dl ($p<0.05$), respectively. The reduction rate of serum total protein and albumin was 0.821 and 0.933, respectively.

Fig. 2 shows the mean levels of serum total protein and albumin concentration before and after DFPP with 12.5% albumin solution as supplementation fluid in 7 DFPPs of 5 patients. The mean serum total protein decreased significantly from 5.77 to 5.22 g/dl ($p<0.05$) but the mean serum albumin elevated from 4.40 to 4.61 g/dl. This elevation of serum albumin was not a significant change. The rate of change serum total protein and albumin was 0.905 and 1.054, respectively.

The reduction rates of IgG and IgM in DFPP treatment with 7.5% albumin solution were 39.8% and 43.6%, and those in DFPP treatment with 12.5% were 38.8% and 42.6%, respectively. In both concentrations of albumin solution, the reduction rates of IgG and IgM were almost the same and not significantly different.

We monitored the continuous changes of the blood volume by optic continuous hematocrit monitor attached in the circuit of DFPP.

In Fig. 3, the abbreviation of minus ΔBV% means the degree of concentrated blood volume estimated by change of hematocrit. The representative two cases were exhibited. During the treatment of DFPP with 7.5% albumin solution, ΔBV% decreased more than minus 20%, while during the treatment of DFPP with 12.5% albumin solution ΔBV% was sustained less than minus 5%.

In the concentration of 7.5% albumin solution as supplementation fluid, hypotension occurred very frequently in the half cases, but in the concentration of 12.5% albumin solution hypotension due to DFPP disappeared (Table 1). In the concentration of 7.5% albumin solution, other clinical complications, such as internal shunt occlusion, fall down to floor, headache and general fatigue, occurred in the rate from 12.5% to 25.0%. In

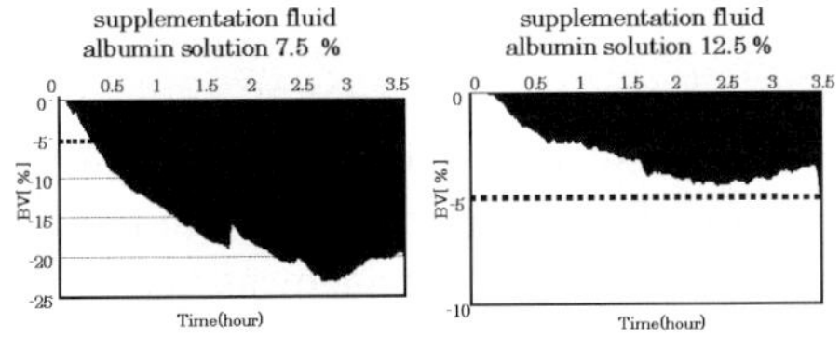

Fig. 3. Intravascular dehydration during DFPP treatment.

Table 1
Complications associated with the treatment of DFPP

Supplementation fluid, 7.5% albumin solution	n=8
Hypotension (SBP <90 mm Hg)	4 (50.0%)
Internal shunt occlusion after DFPP	1 (12.5%)
Fall down after DPFF	1 (12.5%)
Headache	1 (12.55)
General fatigue	2 (25.0%)
Supplementation fluid, 12.5% albumin solution	n=7
Hypotension (SBP <90 mm Hg)	0 (0.0%)

contrast, those complications did not seem to occur in the concentration of 12.5% albumin solution as supplementation fluid.

3. Discussion

In ABO-incompatible kidney transplantation, the higher levels of anti-A or anti-B blood type antibody predict the risk of acute humoral rejection just after the graft operation [5,6]. In order to prevent the acute humoral rejection, antibody removal treatment before transplant operation is an essential method. Usually 2 or 3 treatments must be performed according to the levels of anti-blood type antibody before graft operation.

Plasma exchange is one of the methods of antibody removal treatments. This method requires much fresh frozen plasma (FFP) during the treatment. When we use FFP, the various risks, such as unknown viral infection, allergic reaction and the side effect of citric acid toxicity, are inevitable [7]. Therefore, this method is the undesirable one in view of safety, even though the efficacy for antibody removal is enough.

Hemoadsorption with Biosynsorb column was a highly safe and effective method as antibody removal treatment [8–10]. This column contained artificial carbohydrate antigens corresponding to blood type A or B antigen that were coated on the surface of small silica beads. Biosynsorb could absorb anti-A or anti-B blood type antigens specifically from the circulating blood of recipients, thus, immunoglobulins and other serum proteins did not show the significant alteration after the treatment of antibody removal treatment with Biosynsorb. Since the commercial supply of Biosynsorb has discontinued in recent years, it is not available so far in our country.

As a practical selection, DFPP has been compelled to be a standard method as antibody removal treatment before ABO-incompatible kidney transplantation. DFPP requires supplementation fluid at the operation. The second filter of DFPP removes the fraction of immunoglobulins and at the same time that of albumin from the circulating blood. When we performed DFPP treatment with 7.5% albumin solution as supplementation fluid, we noticed the vivid blood concentration of recipients from the observation by optic continuous monitor attached in the circuit of DFPP (Fig 3). The blood concentration progressing during DFPP treatment was supposed to be interpreted by the decrease of oncotic pressure due to the significant reduction of serum total protein or albumin.

After we raised the albumin solution as supplementation fluid to 12.5%, the extent of blood concentration was sustained in the milder range (Fig. 3). As the interpretation of this alteration, we evaluated serum total protein and albumin concentration before and after

DFPP treatment in both conditions of albumin solution as supplementation fluid (Figs. 1 and 2). Especially in the condition of 12.5% albumin solution, the serum concentration of albumin did not significantly change through DFPP treatment. We considered this fact could prevent adverse effects, such as hypotension, internal shunt occlusion, fall down, etc., that was supposed to be related with intravascular dehydration due to the decrease of plasma oncotic pressure during DFPP treatment (Table 1). Mineshima et al. also reported that inadequate infusion of albumin solution in DFPP treatment might lead to hypoproteinemic symptoms such as edema [11,12]. Like these patients' condition should be the hamper for the safety transplant operation.

From our results, we confirmed DFPP with 12.5% albumin solution as supplementation fluid was safe and effective method for the success of ABO-incompatible kidney transplantation.

References

[1] A. Humpe, et al., Hepatitis C virus transmission through quarantine fresh-frozen plasma, Thromb. Haemost. 84 (2000) 784–788.
[2] Matsubayashi, et al., Transfusion-transmitted hepatitis E caused by apparently indigenous hepatitis E virus strain in Hokkaido, Japan, Transfusion 44 (2004) 934–940.
[3] P. Tardtong, et al., Plasmapheresis for the preparation of HIV free cryoprecipitate, Southeast Asian J. Trop. Med. Public Health 24 (Suppl. 1) (1993) 195–197.
[4] M. Mineshima, et al., Optimum albumin concentration of supplementation fluid for double filtration plasmapheresis, Artif. Organs 16 (1992) 510–513.
[5] H. Ishida, et al., Therapeutic apheresis therapy for ABO-incompatible renal transplantations, Ther. Apher. Dial. 7 (2003) 520–528.
[6] H. Shimmura, et al., Removal of anti-A/B antibodies with plasmapheresis in ABO-incompatible kidney transplantation, Ther. Apher. 4 (2000) 395–398.
[7] D.D. Kiprov, et al., Adverse reactions associated with mobile therapeutic apheresis: analysis of 17,940 procedures, J. Clin. Apher. 16 (2001) 130–133.
[8] T. Agishi, et al., Immunoadsorption of anti-A or anti-B antibody for successful kidney transplantation between ABO incompatible pairs and its limitation. Japanese Biosynsorb Research Group, ASAIO Trans. 37 (1991) M496–M498.
[9] L.M. Sakhrani, et al., Safety and efficacy of BIOSYNSORB immunoadsorption column treatment, Transplant. Proc. 24 (1992) 1735–1737.
[10] T. Agishi, et al., Comparative evaluation of immunoadsorption and double filtration plasmapheresis for removal of anti-A or -B antibody in ABO-incompatible kidney transplantation. Japanese Biosynsorb Research Group, Transplant. Proc. 24 (1992) 557–558.
[11] M. Mineshima, et al., Continuous monitoring of blood volume in double filtration plasmapheresis, ASAIO J. 44 (1998) M465.
[12] M. Mineshima, et al., Optimum albumin concentration of supplementation fluid for double filtration plasmapheresis, Artif. Organs 16 (1992) 510–513.

Rituximab

ELSEVIER

International Congress Series 1292 (2006) 99–104

www.ics-elsevier.com

Newly developed preconditioning regimen consisting of rituximab, splenectomy and plasmapheresis for non-responders to conventional regimen in ABO-incompatible kidney transplantation

Satoshi Teraoka*, Koutaro Kai, Kazuhiro Iwato, Youjiro Kato, Kouji Nanmoku, Akihito Sannomiya, Ichiro Koyama, Tamotsu Toujinbara, Ichiro Nakajima, Shohei Fuchinoue

Tokyo Women's Medical University, Kidney Center, Department of Surgery, 8-1 Kawada-Cho, Shinjuku-Ku, Tokyo, 162-8666, Japan

Abstract. To enable successful ABO-incompatible kidney transplantation, reducing anti-donor blood-type antibody titer to below 1:16 just before the transplantation is considered to be indispensable. We performed successful ABO-incompatible kidney transplantation using new preconditioning regimen, consisting of rituximab, pretransplant splenectomy and plasmapheresis (PP) in 7 cases of non-responders to pretransplant PP. Rituximab was administered intravenously at a dose of 375 mg/M^2 weekly for 2–4 weeks, followed by laparoscopic splenectomy and 4 consecutive sessions of PP. The titer of anti-donor blood type antibody was reduced after PP and was below 1:8–1:16 on the day of the transplantation. CD19$^+$ B cell rapidly decreased to below 1% in the peripheral blood samples and no B cell zone was found in spleen specimen, while CD79$^+$ cell (plasma cell) was observed abundantly in the spleen. One case developed severe neutropenia with high fever probably due to cytomegalovirus (CMV) antigenemia and/or streptococcal bacteremia following twice infusion of rituximab, and both of which were resolved and kidney transplantation was done successfully. No other serious adverse effect was encountered except only one episode of cellular rejection and CMV antigenemia in two cases. Otherwise posttransplant course was smooth in all 7 cases. The kidney grafts were functioning well in all 7 cases during the observation period (13–44 months). © 2006 Published by Elsevier B.V.

Keywords: Kidney transplantation; Rituximab; ABO-incompatible; Anti-blood type antibody; Plasmapheresis

* Corresponding author. Tel./fax: +81 3 5269 7444.
E-mail address: teraoka@kc.twmu.ac.jp (S. Teraoka).

0531-5131/ © 2006 Published by Elsevier B.V.
doi:10.1016/j.ics.2006.03.061

1. Introduction

Kidney transplantation across the ABO-blood type barrier has been enabled by decreasing anti-blood type antibody titer by plasmapheresis (PP) and splenectomy and by the evolution of immunosuppressants [1]. ABO-incompatible kidney transplantation has accounted for 10–15% of live donor kidney transplantation and has been increasing year by year in Japan, which compensated for the organ shortage. In the successful ABO-incompatible kidney transplantation, it is empirically considered indispensable to reduce the anti-donor blood type antibody titer to under 1:16 just before the transplantation [2]. In some cases, however, the anti-donor blood type antibody titer cannot be reduced to 1:16 even after the intensive PP (non-responder), in which kidney transplantation from the concerned donor must be resigned, and other ABO-compatible donor must be provided, otherwise kidney transplantation in itself must be resigned.

Recently anti-CD20 monoclonal antibody, rituximab, was developed and applied to B cell lymphoma [3]. All pre-B cells, and immature and mature B cells express CD20 on their surface membrane so that rituximab eliminates those precursor cells of antibody generating plasma cells by means of complement-dependent cytotoxicity and antibody-dependent cell-mediated cytotoxicity [4–6]. Rituximab, therefore, was considered effective to eliminate the precursor cell of plasma cells, which generated anti-blood type antibodies. We devised new preconditioning regimen consisting of the treatment rituximab, splenectomy and PP for those in which anti-donor blood type antibodies are not reduced to 1:16 even after 4 to 5 sessions of the preoperative PP (non-responder) [7]. Here, we report 7 cases of successful ABO-incompatible kidney transplantation treated with newly developed preconditioning regimen consisting of rituximab, preoperative splenectomy and PP.

2. Patients and methods

Seven cases of ABO-incompatible kidney transplantation were performed by using newly developed preconditioning regimen consisting of rituximab, preoperative splenectomy and PP. Six cases were resistant to 4 to 5 consecutive sessions of PP, while in case 7 the titer of anti-blood type antibody was extremely high, 1:2048, so that rituximab was used from the beginning. Gender, age and original disease of recipients and blood type of recipients and donors were shown in Table 1.

All seven patients were treated with rituximab, anti-CD20 monoclonal antibody, at a dose of 375 mg/M^2 weekly for 2 to 4 weeks. One week before the kidney transplantation,

Table 1
Gender, age and original disease of recipients and blood type of recipients and donors

Case	Gender	Original disease	Recipient blood type	Donor blood type	Remarks
1	M	Alport syndrome	O	A1	Non-responder
2	F	CGN	A	B	Non-responder
3	F	CGN	O	A1	Non-responder
4	M	Diabetic nephropathy	O	A1	Non-responder post-SPK
5	M	CGN	O	A	Non-responder
6	F	IgA	B	AB	Non-responder
7	F	PCK	O	B	High titer 1:2048

Table 2
Observation period, graft function, current serum creatinine level, rejection episode and complications

Case	Follow-up period	Graft function	Current sCr (mg/dl)	Rejection episode	Adverse effect/complication
1	44	Functioning	1.8	Yes (cellular)	CMV Ag-emia
2	41	Functioning	1.3	No	No
3	39	Functioning	1.5	No	No
4	38	Functioning	1.3	No	No
5	37	Functioning	1.5	No	No
6	35	Functioning	0.9	No	No
7	13	Functioning	1.1		Pancytopenia CMV Ag-emia

laparoscopic splenectomy was done and 1 day after the splenectomy, 4 consecutive sessions of double filtration plasmapheresis (DFPP) were done using 5–7% albumin solution as a substitution fluid.

The kidney transplantation was done using the standard procedure after confirming the titer of anti-donor blood type antibody under 1:16, while the donor nephrectomy was done by laparoscopic technique. The immunosuppressive regimen consisted of tacrolimus (Tac) or cyclosporine (CsA), mycophenolate mofetil (MMF), methlypredniso-lone (MPS) and anti-lymphocyte globulin (ALG) (cases 1–3) or basiliximab (cases 4–7). Tac was given at a dose of 0.12 mg/kg initially, and thereafter adjusted to the turget blood trough ranging from 10 to 15 ng/ml for the first posttransplant month. In case of CsA, the initial dose was 8 mg/kg and thereafter dose was adjusted based upon blood C2 level and area under the concentration–time curve (AUC) so as to maintain C2 around 1200 ng/ml and AUC0–4 around 2500 ng/h/ml for the first posttransplant month. MMF was given at a dose of 2000 mg/day for the first posttransplant month, and blood trough level and AUC0–4 were monitored so as to maintain trough level within 1 to 4 μg/ml, and AUC0–4 within 20 to 45 μg/h/ml. MPS was started at a dose of 500 mg/day and was rapidly tapered down to 8 mg/day. In cases 1–3, 20 mg/kg/day of ALG was given intravenously for 14 nbsp;days, while in cases 4–7, 20 mg/day of baisiliximab was given intravenously on day 0 and 4. In case of rejection episode, 500 mg/day of MPS was given intravenously for 2 days and thereafter rapidly tapered to the previous dose.

The titer of anti-blood type A or B immunoglobulin (Ig) was measured by the saline agglutination method for IgM and by the indirect Coomb's test for IgG. The incidence of $CD4^+$, $CD8^+$, $CD25^+$, $CD19^+$, $CD14^+$ and $CD56^+$ in the peripheral blood was monitored by flow cytometry. The extirpated spleen specimen was stained with hematoxylin–eosin (H&E) and with anti-human CD20, CD79 and CD3 monoclonal antibody by immuno-histochemical method. The biopsy specimen of kidney graft was stained with H&E, Masson-trichrome and C4d antibody.

3. Results

Posttransplant course was smooth in all 7 patients for 13 to 44 posttransplant months and current serum creatinine level was between 0.9 and 1.8 mg/dl (Table 2). Acute cellular

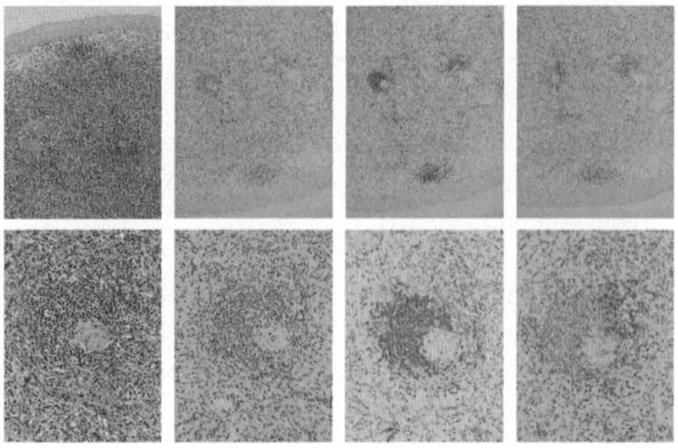

Fig. 1. Histological findings and the distribution of $CD20^+$, $CD79^+$ and $CD3^+$ cells of the extirpated spleen specimen in case 2. Upper row: magnification ×25, lower row: magnification ×100. Immunohistochemical staining with CD20 showed the absence of the B cell zone, while only minimal number of residual B cells were noticed in the T cell zone. Abundant $CD79^+$ plasma cells were observed in the spleen.

rejection episode was observed in only one case (case 1), and no episode of humoral rejection was noticed. Two patients developed cytomegalovirus (CMV) antigenemia (cases 1 and 7). One patient (case 7) developed severe neutropenia and thrombocytopenia 18 days after the second infusion of rituximab associated with sustained high fever and streptococcal bacteremia, which were improved after the treatment with 150–500 μg/day of granulocyte-colony stimulating factor (G-CSF) (for 8 days) and 7.5 g/day of γ-globulin (for 6 days), and platelet infusion (for 3 days). During netropenia, the incidence of $CD3^+CD8^+CD57^+$ in the peripheral blood was 28.2%, and that of $CD3^+CD8^+CD95^+$ was 40.0%. Forty days after the recovery from neutropenia, 4 consecutive sessions of PP were done, followed by successful ABO-incompatible kidney transplantation.

The titer of anti-donor blood type antibody decreased from 1:256–1:2048 to 1:8–1:16, and thereafter it was depressed and ranging from 1:8 to 1:32 after the transplantation. The incidence of:$CD19^+$:B cells in peripheral blood rapidly decreased to less than 1%, and thereafter was depressed within 0 – 1%. The incidence of CD25 in peripheral blood decreased from 17–35% to 0–2% after the twice infusions of basiliximab, and it returned to the previous value 7 to 16 weeks after basiliximab infusion.

Histological findings of the extirpated spleen and the distribution of $CD20^+$, $CD79^+$ and $CD3^+$ cells in the spleen tissue of case 2 were shown in Fig. 1. Immunochemical staining of the extirpated spleen specimen of case 2 showed the absolute absence of the B cell zone and only residual $CD20^+$ B cells in the T cell zone, whereas abundant $CD79^+$ cells, plasma cells, were observed. The histological examination of kidney graft specimen taken on day 8 in case 1 showed no specific finding except only minimal vacuolization of tubular epithelial cells and only slight positive staining of C4d in the basement membrane of peritubular capillaries and glomerular mesangium and capillary basement membrane.

4. Discussion

ABO-incompatible kidney transplantation has been enabled by decreasing anti-blood type antibody titer by PP and splenectomy and by the introduction of potent and selective immunosuppressants [1]. It has been empirically considered indispensable to reduce the titer of anti-donor blood type antibody to under 1 : 16 just before ABO-incompatible kidney transplantation [2], although the permissive minimal titer for the successful ABO-incompatible kidney transplantation has not been identified. In some cases, however, the titer of anti-donor blood type antibody cannot be reduced to 1 : 16 even after the several consecutive sessions of PP, in which kidney transplantation from the concerned donor must be resigned, and other ABO-compatible donor must be provided, otherwise kidney transplantation in itself must be resigned.

Recently developed rituximab is chimeric human-murine anti-CD20 monoclonal antibody and applied to B cell lymphoma [3]. Rituximab effectively eliminates precursor cells of antibody generating plasma cells, namely pre-B cells, and immature and mature B cells which express CD20 on their surface membrane through complement-dependent cytotoxicity and antibody-dependent cell-mediated cytotoxicity [4–6]. Even after the nearly total elimination of B cells, however, antibodies in the serum and plasma cells in the peripheral blood, spleen (Fig. 1) and other lymphoid tissue still remain. These were, we considered, the very reason why PP and splenectomy were required.

The necessity of splenectomy in ABO-incompatible kidney transplantation remains still controversial. The immunohistochemical stain of extirpated spleen specimen showed abundant $CD79^{+}$ cells, plasma cells, in the spleen (Fig. 1), which would be responsible for generating anti-blood type antibodies after the transplantation. Indeed, numerous plasma cells are left intact in other lymphoid tissues, even if plasma cells in spleen are eliminated by the splenectomy. Plasma cells in other lymphoid tissues, however, are considered to decrease in number with time as their precursor cells are eliminated by rituximab. Further investigations are required to elucidate the necessity of splenectomy in ABO-incompatible kidney transplantation.

The dose and the frequency of rituximab administration should be investigated from now on. Additionally the adverse effects of rituximab, especially neutropenia, should be kept in mind. According to data from the Japanese multi-center clinical trial of rituximab, the incidence of neutropenia was 45.9% (72 out of 157 cases), while the incidence of grade 4 neutropenia was 5.7% (9 out of 157 cases). The duration between the treatment with rituximab and the onset of neutropenia was ranging from 1 to 266 days (median: 32.5 days), and the duration between its onset and the recovery was ranging from 1 to 154 days (median: 10 days). With respect to the possible mechanism of rituximab-associated neutropenia, the transient production of autoantibodies directed against neutrophils or their precursors [8], T-lymphocyte-specific cellular response against autologous myeloid precursors [9], apoptosis of mature neutrophils through CD95 (Fas) triggering (probably associated with the induction of T-cell large granular lymphocytes) [10], and myelosuppression mediated by rituximab-induced tumor necrosis factor-α release [11] were reported. In the present study, case 7 developed severe neutropenia and thrombocytopenia 18 days after the second infusion of rituximab which recovered by the treatment with G-CSF and γ-globulin and platelet infusion. In case 7, the incidence of $CD3^{+}CD8^{+}CD57^{+}$ and $CD3^{+}CD8^{+}CD95^{+}$ in peripheral blood was 28.2% and 40.0%, respectively. These suggest that Fas-triggering apoptosis and/or the involvement of T-cell large granular lymphocytes may be related to the pathogenesis of neutropenia in case 7.

References

[1] G.P. Alexandre, et al., Present experiences in series of 26 ABO-incompatible living donor renal allografts, Transplant. Proc. 19 (1987) 4538.
[2] L. Rydberg, ABO-incompatibility in solid organ transplantation, Transfus. Med. 11 (2001) 325.
[3] D.G. Maloney, et al., Phase 1 clinical trial using escalating single-dose infusion of chimeric anti-CD20 monoclonal antibody (IDEC-C2B8) in patients with recurrent B-cell lymphoma, Blood 84 (1994) 2457.
[4] J. Golay, et al., Biologic response of B lymphoma cells to anti-CD20 monoclonal antibody rituximab in vitro: CD55 and CD59 regulate complement-mediated cell lysis, Blood 95 (2000) 3900.
[5] D.G. Maloney, B. Smith, F.R. Applebaum, The anti-tumor effect of monoclonal anti-CD20 antibody (mAb) therapy includes direct anti-proliferative activity and induction of apoptosis in CD20 positive non-Hodgkin's lymphoma (NHL) cell lines, Blood 83 (1996) 637.
[6] M.E. Reff, et al., Depletion of B cells in vivo by a chimeric mouse human monoclonal antibody to CD20, Blood 83 (1994) 435.
[7] T. Sawada, S. Fuchinoue, S. Teraoka, Successful A1-to-O ABO-incompatible kidney transplantation after a preconditioning regimen consisting of anti-CD20 monoclonal antibody infusions, splenectomy and double-filtration plasmapheresis, Transplantation 74 (2002) 1207.
[8] E. Voog, F. Morschhauser, Solal-Celigny, Neutropenia in patients treated with rituximab, N. Engl. J. Med. 348 (2003) 2691.
[9] A.L. Rose, A.M. Forsythe, D.G. Maloney, Agranulocytosis unresponsive to growth factors following rituximab in vivo purging, Blood 101 (2003) 4225.
[10] T. Papadaki, et al., Rituximab-associated immune myelopathy, Blood 102 (2003) 1557.
[11] J. Bienvenu, et al., Tumor necrosis factor alpha release is a major biological event associated with rituximab treatment, Hematol. J. 2 (2001) 378.

ELSEVIER

International Congress Series 1292 (2006) 105–109

www.ics-elsevier.com

Prophylactic use of anti-CD20 monoclonal antibody in ABO-incompatible liver transplantation

Mikiko Ueda *, Atsushi Yoshizawa, Hironori Haga, Fumitaka Oike, Hiroto Egawa, Koichi Tanaka

Department of Transplantation and Immunology, Kyoto University Graduate School of Medicine, 54 Kawara-cho, Shogoin, Sakyo-ku, Kyoto 606-8507, Japan

Abstract. Local infusion of immunosuppression via portal vein catheter and/or hepatic arterial catheter combined with splenectomy has been shown an effective therapy to prevent fatal humoral rejection in ABO-incompatible living donor liver transplantation (LDLT). However, portal vein thrombosis and frequent infectious complications were the significant adverse effects. In this series, anti-CD20 monoclonal antibody (Rituximab) was introduced in stead of portal vein infusion and splenectomy and the efficacy and the timing of Rituximab administration combined with hepatic arterial infusion was examined in 18 patients with the age range of 16 to 68 years (rescue treatment: $n=3$, preemptive treatment: $n=3$, prophylactic treatment: $n=12$) with ABO-incompatible LDLT. Fatal humoral rejection occurred in 2 out of 3 patients with rescue treatment and in 1 out or 3 patients with preemptive treatment, while fatal rejection did not occur in 12 patients with the prophylactic treatment. The frequency of humoral rejection was low (25%) and all humoral rejections ($n=3$) were treatable in the prophylactic treatment. The prophylactic use of Rituximab was markedly effective in ABO-incompatible LDLT.

Keywords: Living donor liver transplantation; ABO-incompatible transplantation; Humoral rejection; Immunosuppression; Anti-CD20 monoclonal antibody

1. Introduction

In Japan, living donor liver transplantation (LDLT) across ABO blood group occupies 8% of the whole LDLT [1] because the selective option of the donors is extremely limited. Once humoral rejection occurs, the grafts are highly lost by rapidly progressing hepatic

* Corresponding author. Tel.: +81 75 751 4323; fax: +81 75 751 4387.
E-mail address: mikiko@kuhp.kyoto-u.ac.jp (M. Ueda).

0531-5131/
doi:10.1016/j.ics.2006.03.063

necrosis or by gradually progressing cholestatic liver failure [2]. To protect these problems, prostaglandin E1 and steroid administration via portal or hepatic arterial infusion catheter for the first several weeks after transplantation was carried out combined with splenectomy to protect microarterial disseminated intravascular coagulation caused by humoral reaction [3]. This infusion therapy has brought improvement in the graft survival. However, portal vein thrombosis and frequent infectious complications were the adverse effects. As a next step of immunosuppression, we adopted anti-CD20 monoclonal antibody (Rituximab) administration instead of splenectomy, and portal infusion through the portal vein was abandoned. In this report, the efficacy and the timing of the Rituximab were examined.

2. Patients and method

2.1. Patient

From March 2004 to July 2005, 18 adult patients including 3 men and 15 women underwent ABO-incompatible LDLT. Their age ranged from 16 years to 68 years (median: 52 years). Primary diseases are liver cirrhosis due to hepatitis B virus (HBV) (6), liver cirrhosis due to hepatitis C virus (HCV) (4), primary biliary cirrhosis (3) and others. Their donors were husbands (5), mothers (4), sons (4), wives (2), sisters (2) and daughter (1). The combination of blood group of the donors and the recipients were A to O (9), B to O (4), AB to A (3), B to A (1) and AB to O (1).

2.2. Operation

Right lobe liver grafts were transplanted in 17 patients and left lobe graft was transplanted in one patient. Splenectomy was not performed. An 18-gauge catheter was placed in a branch of hepatic artery after the hepatic arterial anastomosis was completed.

2.3. Immunosuppression

To reduce the anti-A or B antibodies to less than $\times 8$, plasma exchange (PE) was carried out preoperatively. As a baseline immunosuppression, FK506 and low dose steroid were administered as described elsewhere. Cyclophosphomide with a dosage of 2 mg/kg was infused for the first 2 weeks and then administered per os to reduce antibody production by the plasma cells. Through the hepatic arterial catheter, 125 mg/day of methylprednisolon (MPD) and 0.01 mg/kg/min of prostaglandin E1 were continuously infused for the first several weeks.

2.4. Rituximab administration

Rituximab was administered in three different time points. In rescue group, 375 mg/mm^2 of Rituximab was infused when humoral rejection was diagnosed by histological examination or when humoral rejection was strongly suspected by the rapid increase in liver enzymes. In preemptive group, Rituximab was infused with the same dosage when the ratio of CD20 increased above 30% after LDLT even when rejection was not suspected following the blood chemistry. In prophylactic group, Rituximab was administered with a same dosage preoperatively.

2.5. Monitoring of humoral rejection

Blood chemistry was tested everyday and anti-A or B antibody titers were evaluated everyday or every other day within the first month. The ratios of CD20 and CD19 were evaluated twice a week within the first month. Deterioration of liver function test combined with increase in anti-A or B titers above × 128 or with an increase in the ratio of CD20 or CD19 above 30% was considered as a sign of humoral rejection and the liver biopsy was performed to confirm it by the findings reported by Haga et al. [4].

2.6. Treatment of humoral rejection

When humoral rejection was diagnosed or strongly suspected, 10 mg/kg/day of MPD was administered via the hepatic arterial catheter for a couple of days. PE was carried out to reduce antibodies against ABO blood group antigens when the antibody titer amounted to more than × 128.

3. Results

3.1. Rescue therapy

Three patients received rescue therapy. Patient 1, a 50-year-old man with liver cirrhosis due to HBV, underwent ABO-incompatible LDLT (Table 1). Rapid increase in total bilirubin (T-Bil) levels was observed from postoperative day 5 (pod 5) and liver biopsy

Table 1
Occurrence of humoral rejection and the following outcomes in patients treated with Rituximab administration

Patient	Age	Sex	Original disease	Blood type	Humoral rejection
Rescue treatment ($n=3$)					
1	50yo	M	Liver cirrhosis (HBV), HCC	A to O	Yes, died on 14 pod
2	33yo	F	Liver cirrhosis (HBV)	AB to A	Yes, recovered
3	16yo	F	Autoimmune hepatitis	A to O	Yes, died on 13 pod
Preemptive treatment ($n=3$)					
4	57yo	F	Liver cirrhosis (HCV), HCC	AB to A	Yes, die on 42 pod
5	58yo	F	Liver cirrhosis (HCV)	B to O	No
6	68yo	F	Drug induced liver failure	A to O	Yes, recovered
Prophylactic treatment ($n=12$)					
7	29yo	F	Wilson's disease	B to O	Yes, recovered
8	65yo	F	Liver cirrhosis (HCV)	B to A	No
9	58yo	F	Liver cirrhosis (HBV)	A to O	No
10	38yo	F	Liver cirrhosis (HBV)	A to O	No
11	52yo	M	Liver cirrhosis (HBV), HCC	B to O	No
12	61yo	F	Liver cirrhosis (HCV), HCC	A to O	No
13	51yo	F	Polycystic liver	A to O	No
14	56yo	F	Primary biliary cirrhosis	AB to A	Yes, recovered
15	39yo	F	Primary biliary cirrhosis	AB to O	Yes, recovered
16	34yo	F	Alcoholic liver cirrhosis	B to O	No
17	64yo	F	Primary biliary cirrhosis	A to O	No
18	38yo	M	Liver cirrhosis (HBV)	A to O	No

yo: year old, F: female, M: male, HBV: hepatitis B virus, HCV: hepatitis C virus, HCC: hepatocellular carcinoma, pod: postoperative day.

was performed on day 8 when serum aspartate aminotransferase (AST), alanine aminotransferase (ALT) and T-Bil showed 155 IU/l, 408 IU/l and 22 mg/dl, respectively. Following the histological diagnosis of humoral rejection, hepatic arterial administration of MPD with a dosage of 10 mg/kg/day was started from day 8, Rituximab was infused on day 9 and PE was started on day 10. However, liver function further deteriorated due to massive hepatic necrosis with AST levels of 6289 IU/l, ALT levels of 3886 IU/l and T-Bil levels or 17.1 mg/dl. The patient died from liver failure on day 14. Patient 2 was a 33-year-old woman with HBV liver cirrhosis. T-Bil levels started to increase after pod 3 and liver biopsy was performed when AST, ALT and T-Bil showed 58 IU/l, 338 IU/l and 10.4 mg/dl, respectively on day 7. Following the histological diagnosis of humoral rejection, hepatic arterial administration of MPD and Rituximab infusion were added. Blood chemistry improved soon. Patient 3 was a 16-year-old woman with autoimmune hepatitis. T-Bil levels started to increase in the early postoperative days and AST, ALT and T-Bil showed 248 IU/l, 573 IU/l and 24 mg/dl, respectively on day 5 with the rapid decrease in bile discharge from the biliary drainage tube. Humoral rejection was highly suspected and hepatic arterial administration of MPD and Rituximab administration was added without a confirmed diagnosis by histology. On day 6, AST, ALT and T-Bil showed 2985 IU/l, 2867 IU/l and 22.5 mg/dl, respectively. The patient died from liver failure due to massive hepatic necrosis on pod 13.

3.2. Preemptive therapy

Patient 4 was a 57-year-old woman with liver cirrhosis due to HCV accompanied by hepatocellular carcinoma. The ratio of CD20 increased from 17.2% before operation to 43.1% on day 3. On pod 7, liver enzymes deteriorated (AST: 141 IU/l, ALT: 354 IU/l, T-Bil: 17.2 mg/dl) and the anti-B antibody titer also increased up to $\times 128$. Steroid pulse therapy through the hepatic arterial catheter, Rituximab administration and PE were immediately introduced on day 7 and humoral rejection was confirmed histologically on day 16. Instead of these treatments, the liver function and the histology findings did not improve and the patient died on day 42. Patient 5 with liver cirrhosis due to HCV showed increase in the ratio of CD20 from 20.9% before operation to 48.1% on pod 5. Improvement in liver function test ceased on pod 7 (AST: 94 IU/l, ALT: 238 IU/l, T-Bil 13.1 mg/dl). Rituximab was then administered without the deterioration of liver function test and the blood data improved soon after that. Patient 6 received LDLT for drug-induced fulminant liver failure. Since the ratio of CD20 evaluated on pod 3 was high (48.1%), Rituximab was administered on the same day. Histology of the liver showed humoral rejection on pod 9 without the deterioration of liver function test. The patient was discharged from hospital on day 40 with good liver function.

3.3. Prophylactic therapy

Twelve patients were administered Rituximab 2 to 14 days before the ABO-incompatible LDLT. Nine patients showed no humoral rejection, while three patients were diagnosed as having humoral rejection on pod 6. The latter three patients recovered from humoral rejection following steroid pulse therapy through the hepatic arterial catheter with or without PE.

4. Discussion

The efficacy of anti-CD20 monoclonal antibodies (Rituximab) in ABO-incompatible organ transplantation was first reported in renal transplantation [5], in which patients are more susceptible to humoral rejection. In ABO-incompatible LDLT at our hospital, local infusion therapy of steroid and PGE1 through portal vein catheter in former series and through hepatic arterial catheter in recent series combined with splenectomy has been markedly effective for the improvement of patient survival compared with the previous immunosuppressive treatment without local infusion. However, high incidence of portal vein thrombosis and infectious complication were also observed. In this series, portal infusion and splenectomy were abandoned and Rituximab was administered instead. In the rescue treatment of Rituximab, all three patients presented humoral rejection, including two with fatal rejection. In the preemptive treatment in which the Rituximab was administered when the ratio of CD20 increased more than 30% after LDLT with or without deterioration of liver function test. One patient died from humoral rejection, one overcame humoral rejection, and the other one showed no humoral rejection. Therefore the rescue and preemptive treatment could not prevent fatal humoral rejection, while prophylactic use of Rituximab prevented fatal humoral rejection from three patients with confirmed humoral rejection, and was effective to protect 9 patients from humoral rejection. With these preliminary results, prophylactic use of Rituximab in ABO-incompatible LDLT was markedly effective to protect liver grafts from humoral rejection. The effect of Rituximab administration on infectious complication has to be clarified in the future.

Acknowledgements

This work was supported in part by a Grant-in-Aid for Scientific Research from the Ministry of Education, Culture, Sports, Science and Technology, and for Research on Human Genome, Tissue Engineering Food Biotechnology, Health Sciences Research Grants, from Ministry of Health, Labour and Welfare of Japan.

References

[1] The Japanese Liver Transplantation Society, Liver transplantation in Japan—registry by the Japanese Liver Transplantation Society, Japanese Journal of Transplantation 39 (2004) 634–642.

[2] H. Egawa, et al., Impact of recipient age on outcome of ABO-incompatible living-donor liver transplantation, Transplantation 77 (2004) 403–411.

[3] M. Tanabe, et al., Intraportal infusion therapy as a novel approach to adult ABO-incompatible liver transplantation, Transplantation 73 (2002) 1959–1961.

[4] H. Haga, et al., Periportal edema and necrosis as diagnostic histological features of early humoral rejection in ABO-incompatible liver transplantation, Liver Transplantation 10 (2004) 16–27.

[5] T. Sawada, S. Fuchinoue, S. Teraoka, Successful A1- to O ABO-incompatible kidney transplantation after a preconditioning regimen consisting of anti-CD20 monoclonal antibody infusions, splenectomy, and double-filtration plasmapheresis, Transplantation 74 (2002) 1207–1210.

Sensitization and preformed antibody-positive transplantation

International Congress Series 1292 (2006) 113–119

ELSEVIER

www.ics-elsevier.com

Overcoming antibody barriers to transplantation: ABO-incompatible and positive cross-match kidney transplantation at Mayo Clinic – Rochester

Mark D. Stegall *

Department of Surgery, Division of Transplant, Von Leibig Transplant Center, Mayo Clinic College of Medicine 200 First Street SW, Rochester, MN, 55906 USA

Abstract. Over the past several years, protocols have been developed to allow patients with antibody against either donor blood group (ABO-incompatible) or donor HLA antigens (positive cross-match) to undergo successful kidney transplantation. Important factors determining the development of hyperacute rejection, humoral rejection and long-term graft survival have been defined. In this review, the clinical experience with ABO-incompatible and positive cross-match kidney transplantation at Mayo Clinic, Rochester are described with an emphasis on both patient management issues and gaps in our current knowledge in this emerging field.

Keywords: Donor-specific alloantibody; DSA; Living donor kidney transplantation (LDKTx)

1. Introduction

Kidney transplantation has emerged as the most effective treatment for end-stage renal disease. Compared with dialysis, it results in greater patient survival, improved quality of life, and is cost-effective. Compared with deceased donor transplantation, living donor kidney transplantation (LDKTx) has additional advantages of possibly avoiding dialysis in addition to improved patient and graft survival.

Unfortunately, some patients with an otherwise suitable living donor do not undergo LDKTx because of the presence of antibody to the donor (either anti-blood group or anti-HLA donor-specific alloantibodies, DSA). Historically, because of the risk of

Abbreviations: DSA, donor-specific alloantibody; LDKTx, living donor kidney transplantation.

* Corresponding author.
E-mail address: stegall.mark@mayo.edu.

doi:10.1016/j.ics.2006.03.057

hyperacute rejection or humoral rejection early after engraftment, these antibodies have been considered an absolute contraindication to KTx. Currently, the options for these patients are: 1) be placed on the deceased donor waiting list; 2) enter into a paired living donor program; or 3) undergo a "desensitization" protocol, and receive the living donor kidney despite the presence of anti-donor antibody [1].

Being placed on the deceased donor waiting list is the most commonly used option. However, since most ABO-incompatible candidates are blood group O, their current mean waiting time for a deceased donor kidney is approximately 5 years in the United States. This translates into increased morbidity and mortality both pre- and post-transplant especially in older patients and those with diabetes. In countries with a paucity of deceased donors (such as Japan), they likely will never receive a kidney transplant. Similarly, patients possessing anti-HLA antibodies with a wide range of specificities may never achieve a negative cross-match against any deceased donor. In the USA, more than 8000 patients on the deceased-donor waiting list have a panel reactive antibody greater than 80%, and fewer than 500 are transplanted each year—40% requiring a 0-mismatch kidney donor [2,3].

A second option for these patients is to enter into a paired living donation program. Recently, these "exchange" schemas have been demonstrated to increase the transplantation rate of both ABO-incompatible and sensitized patients. These programs appear especially attractive for candidates with high levels of alloantibody [4,5]. However, these programs have developed relatively slowly due to logistical and ethical hurdles.

The third option for these candidates is to undergo a desensitization regimen and receive the incompatible LDKTx [6–12]. This has been the major focus of our program since its inception in 1999. The remainder of this manuscript will describe the clinical experience in ABO-incompatible and positive cross-match LDKTx at Mayo Clinic – Rochester, outlining not only the main lessons that we have learned so far, but also important gaps in our current knowledge.

2. Antibody levels at baseline and desensitization

Hyperacute rejection is the major catastrophic outcome that must be avoided in both ABO-incompatible and positive cross-match kidney transplantation. We have found that there are antibody levels below which hyperacute rejection is very rare. We also have used antibody deposition on 30-min postreperfusion biopsies as a marker of unsafe antibody levels. Using these criteria, we have developed the concept of a "safe" level of anti-donor antibody. While the exact level appears to vary slightly, we have demonstrated that an anti-blood group isohemagglutination titer of $<1:8$ [9] and a negative T cell AHG cross-match in patients with primarily anti-Class I antibody [13], both appear to be "safe" at the time of transplantation. Since our early experience demonstrated a high incidence of humoral rejection in O recipients of A2 kidneys, we have not used different criteria for A2 versus non-A2 donors.

Achieving these "safe" levels of antibody can be difficult in some patients. Those who at baseline (prior to any therapy) have high levels of anti-blood group antibody (ex. $>1:512$) and those with a T cell AHG cross-match titer $>1:32$ rarely can be "desensitized" (have anti-donor antibody reduced to safe levels) using our current protocols [13]. Alternatively, some sensitized patients have safe levels of antibody at baseline and thus do not need to undergo pretransplant desensitization. The clearest example of this is a sensitized patient with a negative T cell AHG cross-match and a positive T cell flow cytometric cross-match and no demonstrable Class II antibody by solid phase assays. In our laboratory, this correlates with a channel shift <300 on the T cell flow cross-match. While these patients do not undergo hyperacute rejection, they are at risk for humoral rejection.

There are unsafe levels of anti-Class II that can cause hyperacute rejection and early antibody deposition. This is demonstrated most clearly in patients who have only anti-Class II antibody and no anti-Class I antibody as determined by solid phase assays. However, many sensitized patients have a combination of anti-Class I and anti-Class II antibodies. Since the B cell cross-match is affected by both groups of antibodies (B cells express both Class I and Class II), assessing the level of anti-Class II antibodies using the B cell cross-match assay is unreliable. In our laboratory, there has been a poor correlation between the B cell cytotoxicity cross-match assay and the B cell flow cytometric cross-match assay. While we have successfully transplanted patients with a wide variety of B cell flow cytometric cross-match channel shifts, our current protocols require that at the time of transplantation that the patient have: a) a negative T cell AHG and B cell cytotoxicity cross-matches; and b) both the T and B cell flow cytometric cross-matches have channel shifts <300. This approach has avoided hyperacute in all but 1 of the last 54 sensitized recipients.

The two major approaches to desensitization in positive cross-match kidney transplant recipients has been multiple plasmapheresis (PP) treatments or high dose intravenous immunoglobulin (IVIG). In a comparative study, we found that while both are effective at reducing DSA levels, PP is slightly more successful and reproducible in patients with high level DSA [13]. Some of our early protocols included splenectomy in an effort to reduce antibody-secreting cells and enhance desensitization. However, our recent experience suggests that splenectomy does not enhance desensitization in ABO-incompatible kidney transplant recipients [14]. Mechanistically, the observed resistance to desensitization is most likely due to the general resistance of plasma cells to most agents used in our protocols including anti-CD20 antibody, rabbit anti-thymocyte globulin and high dose intravenous immunoglobulin—at least in the time frame of desensitization.

Early in our experience, we transplanted 10 patients who were able to achieve low titers, (undiluted $-1:8$) but not a completely negative T cell AHG cross-match. Of these 10 patients, 70% developed humoral rejection and allograft loss occurred in 50% (5/10) with two of these due to hyperacute rejection. This experience forms the basis for requiring a negative T cell AHG cross-match at the time of transplantation.

3. Early posttransplant management and humoral rejection

Early after transplantation–especially in the first 2 weeks–the development of acute humoral rejection (AHR) correlates with: (a) the level of anti-donor antibody at baseline, i.e. patients with higher baseline levels have higher AHR rates; (b) anti-donor antibody levels at the time of AHR; for example, ABO-incompatible patients with anti-donor blood group levels >1:32 and sensitized patients with flow cytometric cross-match channel shifts >400 usually have histologic changes of AHR. Mechanistically, it appears likely that the increase in anti-donor antibody in patients who develop AHR after transplant is the result of persistent antibody production by preexisting plasma cells and by the development of new plasma cells resulting from the introduction of donor antigen.

Given these findings, our protocols have evolved to include preemptive PP treatments and antibody monitoring aimed to maintain low levels of anti-donor antibody in the first 2 weeks after transplantation. In ABO-incompatible kidney transplants, the goal is to keep the isoagglutination anti-blood group antibody titer less than 1:16 for 2 weeks. For sensitized patients, the goal is to keep both the T and B cell channel shift less than 300 in the first 2 weeks.

We treat AHR with reinstitution of PP and high dose corticosteroids. When AHR persists despite these treatments, we generally perform splenectomy in an effort to reduce antibody-secreting cells. However, the efficacy of splenectomy is unclear. In contrast to other reports demonstrating an increase in acute cellular rejection in sensitized recipients, the use of rATG in our protocols has resulted in only three cases of acute cellular rejection in 124 patients.

Our current protocols for desensitization and posttransplant management are outlined in Table 1.

Table 1
Desensitization and posttransplant management protocols

ABO-incompatible
Exclude patients with baseline anti-blood group titer >1:512
Daily PP to achieve a titer <1:8 on the day of transplantation
Preemptive PP × 3 days
Monitor titer daily and maintain titer <1:16 for 14 days using PP as needed
Positive cross-match
Exclude patients with baseline T cell AHG cross-match titer >1:32
High level DSA
Defined as a positive T cell AHG cross-match and T and B cell flow cross-match channel shift >300
Daily PP to achieve a channel shift <300 on the day of transplantation (correlates with a negative T cell AHG cross-match)
Preemptive PP × 3 days
Monitor cross-match and protocol biopsies on days 4, 7 and 14 to maintain channel shifts <300 for the first 14 days using PP as needed
Low level DSA
T and B cell flow cross-match channel shift <300
No pretransplant treatment
Monitor cross-match and protocol biopsies on days 4, 7 and 14 to maintain channel shifts <300 for the first 14 days using PP as needed
All patients
Thymoglobulin induction (1.5 mg/kg/day) on days 0, 1, 2, 4 and 6
Maintenance with tacrolimus, mycophenolate mofetil and prednisone

4. Late outcomes

Humoral rejection is rare beyond 2 months posttransplant in both ABO-incompatible and positive cross-match LDKTx recipients. Generally, anti-donor antibody is lower at this point after transplant, and is well tolerated by the allograft. In three instances in which the T cell AHG cross-match has remained positive beyond 1 month after transplant, all three patients developed accelerated transplant glomerulopathy, and lost their grafts in the first year.

Late after transplantation (3 months and beyond), anti-donor antibody levels tend to remain at relatively low levels or even disappear (especially common in sensitized patients) [15,16]. These low levels of antibody appear to be well tolerated by the allograft. Recently, we performed a retrospective review of protocol renal allograft biopsies in these patients [17]. At 1 year after transplantation, the majority of ABO-incompatible and positive cross-match LDKTx recipients had the same minor histologic changes (Banff Ci1 lesions) as observed in conventional KTx recipients [18]. Positive cross-match LDKTx showed an increase in the incidence of transplant glomerulopathy at 1 year. However, the development of transplant glomerulopathy correlated with a prior acute humoral rejection episode but not with the persistence of DSA.

5. Summary of clinical outcomes at Mayo Clinic – Rochester

We have performed 62 ABO-incompatible LDKTx at Mayo Clinic – Rochester as of 1/1/2006 including 13 A2 donors. A recent analysis of the first 40 recipients showed a 1-year patient survival of 95.0% (Fig. 1). This compared well with the 97% patient survival in a cohort of 77 non-sensitized ABO-compatible patients ($p = 0.29$).

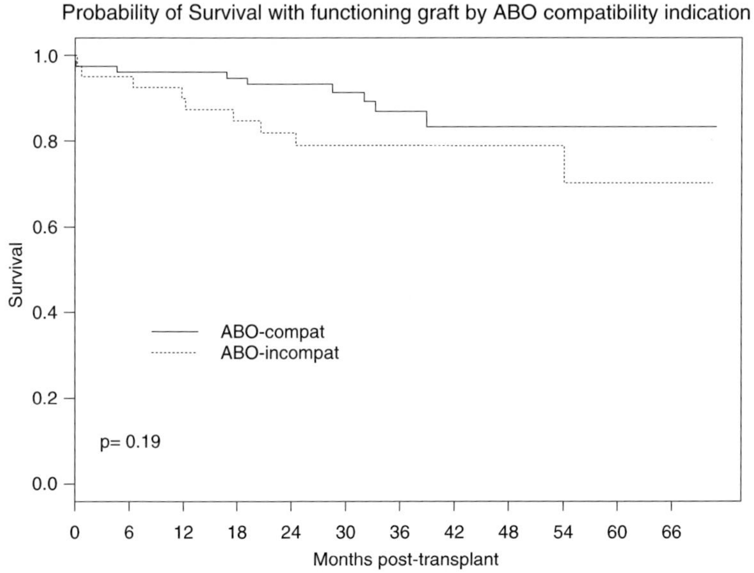

Fig. 1. Probability of survival with functional graft by ABO compatibility indication.

The incidence of humoral rejection in the ABO-incompatible group was 30%. The 1-year death-censored graft survival was 96% in the ABO-compatible group and 90% in the ABO-incompatible group. Graft survival did not differ significantly between the two groups ($p=0.19$). Four ABO-incompatible kidneys failed within the first year, one due to early persistent humoral rejection, two because of accelerated glomerulopathy and chronic allograft nephropathy, and one secondary to a renal artery pseudoaneurysm. The mean serum creatinine was similar at 1 year in the ABO-incompatible and ABO-compatible groups (1.58+0.58 mg/dl vs. 1.69+0.03 mg/dl, respectively).

As of 1/1/2006 we have performed 124 positive cross-match living donor kidney transplants including 78 with high level DSA and 45 with low level DSA at baseline. Of these patients, 36 (46%) of the high level DSA patients and 7 (16%) of the low level DSA patients were treated for humoral rejection. In a recent analysis of patients with high level DSA at baseline, the overall 1-year actuarial patient survival was 93% and the 1-year actuarial graft survival was 82% (follow-up of 127–1915 days). At 6 months, the serum creatinine in the patients who achieved desensitization, underwent transplant and still had a functioning graft was 1.51+0.58 mg/dl. The 1-year actuarial patient and graft survival for low level DSA is 95% and 90%, respectively.

6. The future

A major barrier to the widespread application of both ABO-incompatible and positive cross-match kidney transplantation is the increased cost compared with conventional transplants. We recently performed a retrospective study comparing 40 ABO-incompatible with 77 matching ABO-compatible living donor renal allografts with respect to complications, resource utilization and cost from day − 14 to 90 days after transplantation. Overall, surgery-related complications and resource utilization were increased in the ABO-incompatible group, primarily due to the desensitization protocol and antibody-mediated rejection. In the absence of rejection, the mean number of complications was similar for both groups. ABO-incompatible kidney transplantation was approximately $38,000 more expensive than ABO-compatible transplants, but was cost effective when compared with maintaining the patient on dialysis while waiting for a blood group-compatible deceased donor kidney.

Some of the major gaps in our knowledge in this field include a general paucity of understanding of the mechanisms of antibody production by plasma cells and methods to control them. In addition, we have a very poor understanding of the molecular mediators of acute humoral rejection including not only the role of complement activation but also of possible complement-independent mechanisms such as endothelial cell activation and apoptosis. Finally, mechanisms of enhancing long-term allograft survival—involving the late disappearance of antibody or the development of resistance to antibody by the graft (termed accommodation) [19] have been studied in only a few experimental models and rarely in humans.

7. Conclusion

Both ABO-incompatible and positive cross-match kidney transplantation have shown remarkable success over the past several years offering the possibility of transplantation to an increasing number of patients with end-stage renal disease. However, significant problems remain such as the inability to desensitize all patients and the risk of early humoral rejection with its associated increase in both immediate and late graft loss. Future research efforts focusing on the mechanisms of antibody production and its impact on the graft should provide for continued progress in this new and difficult field.

References

[1] M.D. Stegall, P.G. Dean, J.M. Gloor, ABO-incompatible kidney transplantation, Transplantation 78 (5) (2004) 635–640.

[2] www.unos.org accessed 26 November 2005.

[3] M.D. Stegall, et al., Organ Procurement and Transplantation Network/United Network for Organ Sharing Kidney/Pancreas Transplantation Committee. Survival of mandatorily shared cadaveric kidneys and their paybacks in the zero mismatch era, Transplantation 74 (2002) 670–675.

[4] D.L. Segev, et al., Kidney paired donation and optimizing the use of live donor organs, JAMA 293 (2005) 1883–1890.

[5] R.A. Montgomery, et al., Clinical results from transplanting incompatible live donor kidney donor/recipient pairs using kidney paired donation, JAMA 294 (2005) 1663–1665.

[6] K. Tanabe, et al., Long-term results of ABO-incompatible living kidney transplantation, Transplantation 65 (1998) 224–228.

[7] E. Schweitzer, et al., A high panel-reactive antibody rescue protocol for cross-match-positive live donor kidney transplants, Transplantation 70 (10) (2000) 1531.

[8] R.A. Montgomery, et al., Plasmapheresis and intravenous immune globulin provides effective rescue therapy for refractory humoral rejection and allows kidneys to be successfully transplanted into cross-match-positive recipients, Transplantation 70 (6) (2000) 887.

[9] J.M. Gloor, et al., ABO-incompatible kidney transplantation using both A2 and non-A2 living donors, Transplantation 75 (7) (2003) 971–977.

[10] J.M. Gloor, et al., Overcoming a positive crossmatch in living donor kidney transplantation, Am. J. Transp. 3 (8) (2003) 1017.

[11] S.C. Jordan, et al., Intravenous immune globulin treatment inhibits crossmatch positivity and allows for successful transplantation of incompatible organs in living-donor and cadaver recipients, Transplantation 76 (4) (2003) 631.

[12] D. Glotz, et al., Desensitization and subsequent kidney transplantation of patients using intravenous immunoglobulin, Am. J. Transp. 2 (2002) 758.

[13] M.D. Stegall, J. Gloor, J.L. Winters, S.B. Moore, DeGoey, A comparison of plasmapheresis vs high-dose IVIG desensitization in renal allograft recipients with high levels of donor specific alloantibody, Am. J. Transplant 6 (2) (2006) 346–351.

[14] J.M. Gloor, et al., A comparison of splenectomy versus intensive posttransplant antidonor blood group antibody monitoring without splenectomy in ABO-incompatible kidney transplantation, Transplantation 80 (2005) 1572–1577.

[15] A.A. Zachary, et al., Specific and durable elimination of antibody to donor HLA antigens in renal transplant patients, Transplantation 76 (10) (2003) 1519.

[16] J.M. Gloor, et al., Persistence of low levels of alloantibody after desensitization in crossmatch positive living donor kidney transplantation, Transplantation 78 (2) (2003) 221.

[17] J.M. Gloor, M.D. Stegall, F.C. Cosio, et al. Histologic findings in renal allografts one-year after positive crossmatch or ABO incompatible kidney transplantation, in press.

[18] F.G. Cosio, et al., Predicting subsequent decline in kidney allograft function from early surveillance biopsies, Am. J. Transp. 5 (2005) 2464–2472.

[19] W.D. Park, et al., Accommodation in ABO-incompatible kidney allografts, a novel mechanism of self-protection against anti body-mediated injury, Am. J. Transp. 3 (2003) 952–960.

Xenotransplantation

International Congress Series 1292 (2006) 123–127

www.ics-elsevier.com

GalT knockout pig to baboon xenotransplantation

Kazuhiko Yamada *, David H. Sachs

Transplantation Biology Research Center, Department of Surgery, Massachusetts General Hospital and Harvard Medical School, MGH-East; 13th Street, CNY-149, 9019, Boston, MA 02129, USA

Abstract. The success and widespread acceptance of clinical allotransplantation has led to a shortage of cadaveric organs and a resurgence of interest in xenotransplantation. Although swine are generally regarded as the preferred source of xenogeneic organs, the severe immunologic response to swine organs has so far precluded their clinical use. However, we have recently obtained pigs not expressing the alpha 1,3-galactosyltransferase gene (GalT-KO swine). We have reported initial results using GalT-KO swine as donors to baboons which demonstrated survival of a life-supporting renal graft for up to 83 days without rejection when combined with a regimen designed to induce tolerance by vascularized donor thymic grafts. Although further improvements will be needed to warrant a clinical trial of xenotransplantation, the initial results are encouraging. In addition to genetic modification of donor pigs, it is hoped that our tolerance-inducing regimen will allow successful clinical xenotransplantation by overcoming additional xenogeneic immunological barriers.

Keywords: Xenotransplantation; Tolerance; α-1,3-Galactosyltransferase knockout; Miniature swine

1. Introduction

The shortage of donors for patients in need of organ transplants continues to be a health care crisis. Donor organs from other species are abundant, but their incompatibility in humans has precluded their use thus far. Therefore, as a continuation of our previous work, we have attempted to address the organ shortage by transplanting porcine organs as discordant xenografts to nonhuman primates. Until recently, the rejection caused by anti-Gal natural antibodies (anti-Gal Nab) in baboons has been a major barrier to the research of pig-to-baboon xenograft tolerance because these antibodies caused overwhelming rejection, either immediately (HAR) or, when other manipulations were utilized, in a

* Corresponding author. Tel.: +1 617 726 8029; fax: +1 617 726 4067.
E-mail address: kaz.yamada@tbrc.mgh.harvard.edu (K. Yamada).

0531-5131/ © 2006 Published by Elsevier B.V.
doi:10.1016/j.ics.2006.03.062

delayed fashion [1–6]. However, this barrier has been eliminated in the past year through development of a new breed of α-1,3-galactosyltransferase knockout (GalT-KO) MGH miniature swine, which lack the GalT gene [7,8]. Consequently, we may now transplant organs from pigs to primates without the overwhelming rejection caused by antiGal natural antibodies (Nab) in baboons.

2. Tolerance induction as a strategy for successful xenotransplantation

Successful efforts to control HAR, including the elimination of Gal expression on pig cells, exposed the severity of delayed xenograft rejection (DXR) and acute cellular rejection (ACR). In an attempt to control these reactions, many protocols were developed to block various parts of the immune system's response to xenoantigens. The level of immunosuppression needed to prolong xenograft survival was prohibitive, and was associated with significant morbidity and mortality. Additionally, these regimens have not yielded survival times that would merit clinical trials. Given these factors, our lab believes that the induction of tolerance will be necessary for successful xenotransplantation. Thus far, we have attempted two different methods of inducing tolerance to pig antigens, one via mixed chimerism protocols and the other via thymic transplantation.

2.1. Mixed chimerism for the induction of tolerance

Mixed chimerism is achieved by the transplantation of bone marrow or blood progenitor cells, which engraft, leading to the coexistence of donor and recipient hematopoietic cells. When this occurs, the recipient becomes tolerant to donor antigens. This tolerance is thought to take place via a central mechanism in which donor cells migrate to the thymus where they induce clonal deletion of maturing donor-reactive thymocytes [9]. Preexisting donor reactive T cells are nonspecifically deleted by myeloablation or antibody-mediated T cell depletion, or they are specifically inactivated by costimulatory blockade with donor antigens [10,11]. Studies utilizing small animals have shown that this mechanism was active across xenogeneic barriers, and that mixed chimerism was able to prevent HAR, DXR and T cell-mediated rejection of cardiac xenografts in a rat to GalT-KO mouse model [12,13]. However, thus far, investigations into inducing mixed chimerism in a clinically relevant model using pig bone marrow (BM) cells transplanted into nonhuman primates have not been successful. The authors are now attempting to improve these results by utilizing mobilized GalT-KO animals as BM donors. Initial results indicate that much higher levels of chimerism can be attained using this protocol (data not published), but it remains to be seen whether stable mixed chimerism and tolerance induction can be achieved.

2.2. Thymic transplantation for the induction of tolerance

Thymic transplantation is also thought to lead to tolerance by a central or deletional mechanism. Recipient donor reactive T cells are depleted with T cell antibodies prior to thymic transplantation. The naïve recipient cells then migrate to the donor thymus where allo- or xenoreactive T cells are deleted via negative selection. Recipient dendritic cells also migrate to the donor thymus, providing negative selection for autoreactive T cells. T cells active against other antigens seem to mature normally, leading to donor-specific tolerance. Early studies in mice demonstrated that the transplantation of fetal or neonatal pig thymic tissue to thymectomized mice produced tolerance to pig skin grafts [14,15]. However, we have reported that the prevascularization of donor thymic tissue is essential for the induction of tolerance by donor thymi in large animal models [16,17]. When using nonvascularized thymic grafts, there is a significant deterioration of thymic graft architecture during the period of neovascularization [16] that results in negative effects on thymic deletional mechanisms to donor-xenoreactive T cells. Thus, we have developed two methods of transplanting vascularized thymic tissue: direct vascular anastomosis of the thymic blood supply [18], and the transplantation of a thymokidney (prepared by injecting autologous thymic tissue under the renal capsule and allowing 2 months for neovascularization prior to transplantation) [19]. Our studies have demonstrated functional thymopoiesis in transplanted thymic grafts and donor-specific tolerance induction across a full MHC mismatched barrier in an allogeneic miniature swine model [17,20,21].

3. Initial results of tolerance inducing strategies

3.1. hDAF thymokidney transplantation

The success of tolerance induction by the transplantation of vascularized donor thymus across fully allogeneic barriers led us to extend this strategy to pig to baboon xenotransplantation. Initial studies in the pig to baboon model utilized hDAF transgenic swine as the source of thymic tissue or of composite thymokidney grafts [22]. All recipient baboons underwent either preoperative thymectomy or thymic irradiation, in addition to T cell depletion. The thymokidneys functioned for up to 30 days, with evidence of viable thymic epithelium and Hassall's corpuscles in the thymic implants. Despite evidence of donor-specific hyporesponsiveness by in vitro MLR in some animals, the grafts were rejected in a pattern consistent with DXR, probably due to the return of anti-Gal natural antibodies. Since the production of anti-Gal natural antibodies is T cell-independent, T cell-specific tolerance would not prevent rejection by natural antibodies, but would prevent the development of T cell-dependent anti-pig antibodies. It was concluded that the vascularized thymic grafts induced T cell-specific tolerance, but that eventual rejection due to the anti-Gal antibody response could not be overcome.

3.2. GalT-KO vascularized thymus and thymokidney transplantation

By utilizing GalT-KO animals as donors of either vascularized thymic tissue or of thymokidneys we have attained markedly prolonged renal xenograft survival with normal renal function for up to 83 days [23] (Fig. 1A, B) (as compared with the longest survival of only 30 days with hDAF thymokidneys). The longest surviving recipient of a GalT KO thymokidney died of causes other than rejection (myocardial infarct related to the flushing of a misplaced carotid arterial catheter), and histological analysis of the kidney graft showed no evidence of cellular or humoral rejection at the time of death. The immunosuppressive regimens were being tapered in the longest surviving animals. These animals demonstrated pig-specific unresponsiveness in MLRs, and the animal that survived for 83 days demonstrated donor-specific unresponsiveness with normal anti-third-

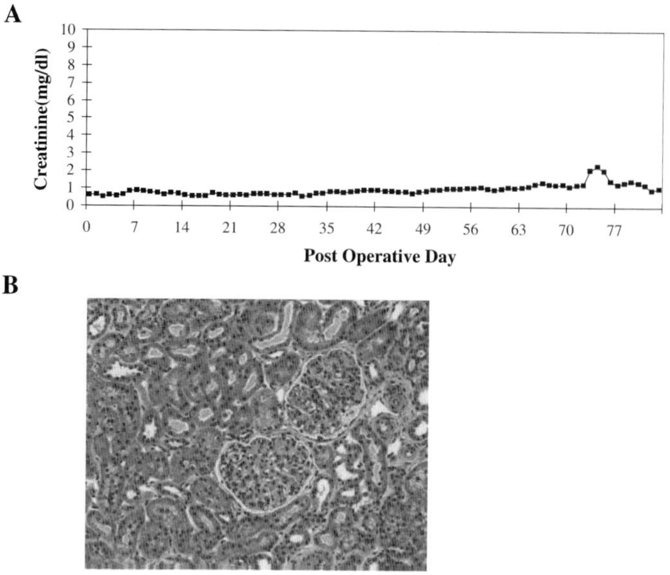

Fig. 1. A baboon recipient of a GalT-KO thymokidney. Creatinine levels following transplantation (A) and thymokidney biopsy on day 60 (B) (H&E).

party allogeneic responses in CTL assays by day 78, suggesting that the baboon was on a path toward tolerance [23]. The lack of histological evidence for rejection and the evidence for tolerance suggest that the immunosuppressive regimen can be decreased in future experiments, with a concomitant decrease in associated morbidity and mortality.

In contrast to the baboons that received a GalT-KO thymus and kidney together, all baboons that received a GalT-KO kidney alone rejected their grafts within 34 days, despite similar immunosuppressive regimens. Histologically, the xenografts displayed interstitial edema as well as mononuclear and polynuclear cell infiltration with interstitial hemorrhage, indicating that both cellular and humoral rejections were involved.

4. Conclusion

In summary, utilizing GalT-KO pigs as donors and a tolerance inducing strategy (i.e. co-transplantation of vascularized thymus), we have kept xenotransplanted primates alive with functioning xenografts for more than 80 days without evidence of rejection. The xenografts functioned in a life-supporting manner, and recipients given minimal immunosuppression in the maintenance phase did not develop sensitization to donors. In the future, we plan to build on this progress using GalT-KO pig donors to identify and surmount further barriers to tolerance, bringing us increasingly close to the goal of making xenotransplantation feasible in the clinical setting. Although clinically applicable xenotransplantation presents a wide range of benefits, the most important benefit is helping patients in end state organ failure who are either unable to tolerate large doses of immunosuppression or for whom there are no compatible organs available due to organ shortage or presensitization to potential donors.

References

[1] A.H. Good, et al., Identification of carbohydrate structures that bind human antiporcine antibodies: implications for discordant xenografting in humans, Transplant. Proc. 24 (1992) 559–562.

[2] D.K.C. Cooper, Depletion of natural antibodies in non-human primates – a step towards successful discordant xenografting in humans, Clin. Transplant. 6 (1992) 178–183.

[3] R. Oriol, et al., Carbohydrate antigens of pig tissues reacting with human natural antibodies as potential targets for hyperacute vascular rejection in pig-to-man organ xenotransplantation, Transplantation 56 (1993) 1433–1442.

[4] M. Cascalho, B.M. Ogle, J.L. Platt, Xenotransplantation and the future of renal replacement, J. Am. Soc. Nephrol. 15 (2004) 1106–1112.

[5] F.H. Bach, et al., Delayed xenograft rejection, Immunol. Today 17 (1996) 379–384.

[6] D.K. Cooper, B. Gollackner, D.H. Sachs, Will the pig solve the transplantation backlog? Annu. Rev. Med. 53 (2002) 133–147.

[7] L. Lai, et al., Production of –1,3-galactosyltransferase knockout pigs by nuclear transfer cloning, Science 295 (2002) 1089–1092.

[8] D. Kolber-Simonds, et al., Production of {alpha}-1,3-galactosyltransferase null pigs by means of nuclear transfer with fibroblasts bearing loss of heterozygosity mutations, Proc. Natl. Acad. Sci. U. S. A. 101 (2004) 7335–7340.

[9] M. Sykes, Mixed chimerism and transplant tolerance, Immunity 14 (2001) 417–424.

[10] N.J. Mueller, et al., Early weaning of piglets fails to exclude porcine lymphotropic herpes virus, Xenotransplant 12 (2005) 59–62.

[11] T. Wekerle, et al., Extrathymic T cell deletion and allogeneic stem cell engraftment induced with costimulatory blockade is followed by central T cell tolerance, J. Exp. Med. 187 (1998) 2037–2044.

[12] H. Ohdan, et al., Mixed chimerism induced without lethal conditioning prevents T cell- and anti-Gal alpha 1,3Gal-mediated graft rejection, J. Clin. Invest. 104 (1999) 281–290.

[13] H. Ohdan, et al., T cell and B cell tolerance to GALalpha1,3GAL-expressing heart xenografts is achieved in alpha1,3-galactosyltransferase-deficient mice by nonmyeloablative induction of mixed chimerism, Transplantation 71 (2001) 1532–1542.

[14] Y. Zhao, et al., Skin graft tolerance across a discordant xenogeneic barrier, Nat. Med. 2 (1996) 1211–1216.

[15] J.I. Rodriguez-Barbosa, et al., Enhanced CD4 reconstitution by grafting neonatal porcine tissue in alternative locations is associated with donor-specific tolerance and suppression of preexisting xenoreactive T cells, Transplantation 72 (2001) 1223–1231.

[16] G.W. Haller, et al., Thymic transplantation across an MHC Class I barrier in swine, J. Immunol. 163 (1999) 3785–3792.

[17] K. Yamada, et al., Thymic transplantation in miniature swine: II. Induction of tolerance by transplantation of composite thymokidneys to thymectomized recipients, J. Immunol. 164 (2000) 3079–3086.

[18] J.C. LaMattina, et al., Vascularized thymic lobe transplantation in miniature swine: I. Vascularized thymic lobe allografts support thymopoiesis, Transplantation 73 (2002) 826–831.

[19] K. Yamada, et al., Thymic transplantation in miniature swine: I. Development and function of the "thymokidney", Transplantation 68 (1999) 1684–1692.

[20] K. Yamada, et al., Thymic transplantation in miniature swine: III. Induction of tolerance by transplantation of composite thymokidneys across fully major histocompatibility complex-mismatched barriers, Transplantation 76 (2003) 530–536.

[21] C. Kamano, et al., Vascularized thymic lobe transplantation in miniature swine: thymopoiesis and tolerance induction across fully MHC-mismatched barriers, Proc. Natl. Acad. Sci. U. S. A. 101 (2004) 3827–3832.

[22] R.N. Barth, et al., Xenogeneic thymokidney and thymic tissue transplantation in a pig-to-baboon model: I. Evidence for pig-specific T-cell unresponsiveness, Transplantation 75 (2003) 1615–1624.

[23] K. Yamada, et al., Marked prolongation of porcine renal xenograft survival in baboons through the use of alpha1,3-galactosyltransferase gene-knockout donors and the cotransplantation of vascularized thymic tissue, Nat. Med. 11 (2005) 32–34.

Author index

Aikawa, A., 8
Asahara, T., 13
Asanuma, H., 42
Azimzadeh, A.M.I., 63

Egawa, H., 25, 105

Fuchinoue, S., 99
Fujishiro, J., 13

Gejyo, F., 91

Haga, H., 25, 105
Hakamata, Y., 13
Hanto, D.W., 53
Hasegawa, A., 8
Hasegawa, S., 91
Hasnizume, K., 13

Inasaka, J., 8
Inoue, S., 13
Itabashi, Y., 8
Iwamoto, S., 13
Iwato, K., 99

Kai, K., 99
Kanai, T., 8
Kaneko, M., 13
Kato, Y., 99
Kawada, N., 8
Kawamura, T., 8
Kobayashi, E., 13
Kobayashi, T., 3
Koyama, I., 99

Manabe, T., 25
Merion, R.M., 63
Miyagawa-Hayashino, A., 25
Mizuiri, S., 8
Moore, J., 63

Nakagawa, Y., 91
Nakajima, I., 99
Nanmoku, K., 99
Nanpo, Y., 42
Nishi, S., 91

Ohdan, H., 13
Oike, F., 105

Pierson, R.N., 63

Sachs, D.H., 123
Saito, K., 35, 91
Sakai, K., 8
Sakashita, H., 25
Saneshige, M., 42
Sannomiya, A., 99
Satoh, H., 42
Shishido, S., 42
Stegall, M.D., 113

Tahara, K., 13
Takahashi, K., v, 35, 73, 91
Takehiro, O., 8
Takeuchi, K., 13
Tanaka, K., 105
Teraoka, S., 99
Toujinbara, T., 99

Ueda, M., 105

Wen, M.-C., 25

Yamada, K., 123
Yamashita, M., 8
Yoshizawa, A., 105

Zhou, W., 13

Keyword index

A/B transferase 13
ABO blood type antigen 13
ABO incompatibility 35
ABO-incompatibility 42, 73
ABO-incompatible 99
ABO-incompatible kidney transplantation 8
ABO-incompatible transplant 63
ABO-incompatible transplantation 3, 53, 105
Accommodation 35, 53, 73
Anti-A/B antibody titer 3
Anti-blood type antibody 99
Antibody-mediated rejection 25, 63, 73
Anti-CD20 monoclonal antibody 105

Blood group antibody 8
Blood group antigen 8

C4d 25
Children 42

Donor-specific alloantibody 113
Double filtration plasma apheresis (DFPP) 91
DSA 113

α-1,3-Galactosyltransferase knockout 123

Heme oxygenase-1 53
Humoral rejection 25, 105
Hyperacute rejection 63, 73
Hypotension 91

Immunosuppression 73, 105
Inter-institutional variation 3
Intravascular dehydration 91

Kidney transplantation 35, 42, 73, 99

Living donor kidney transplantation (LDKTx) 113
Living donor liver transplantation 105
Lung transplant 63

Miniature swine 123

Oncotic pressure 91

Periportal edema and necrosis 25
Plasmapheresis 42, 99
Protective genes 53

Rejection activity index 25
Rituximab 99

Small bowel transplantation 13
Splenectomy 42, 73
Survey 3

Tolerance 123
Transgenic rat 13

Xenotransplantation 123